# The War on Waiting for Hospital Treatment

WHAT HAS LABOUR ACHIEVED AND WHAT CHALLENGES REMAIN?

ANTHONY HARRISON AND JOHN APPLEBY

The King's Fund is an independent charitable foundation working for better health, especially in London. We carry out research, policy analysis and development activities, working on our own, in partnerships, and through funding. We are a major resource to people working in health, offering leadership development programmes; seminars and workshops; publications; information and library services; and conference and meeting facilities.

Published by
King's Fund
11–13 Cavendish Square
London W1G 0AN
www.kingsfund.org.uk

© King's Fund 2005

Charity registration number: 207401

First published 2005

ISBN 1 85717 496 8


Available from:
King's Fund Publications
11–13 Cavendish Square
London W1G 0AN
Tel: 020 7307 2591
Fax: 020 7307 2801
Email: bookshop@kingsfund.org.uk
www.kingsfund.org.uk/publications

Edited by Andrew Ross
Typeset by Grasshopper Design Company
Printed and bound in Great Britain by Hobbs

# Contents

# List of figures

**STATISTICAL SOURCES**

Nearly all the figures in this paper have been constructed from official Department of Health statistics. A variety of the Department's publications and sources were used in compiling the figures showing trends – for example, statistical bulletins and web-based material – and so the source is given as 'Department of Health Statistics'. Where only one source has been used, this source is referenced.

# About the authors

**Anthony Harrison**

Anthony Harrison is a Fellow in Health Policy at the King's Fund. Anthony has published extensively on the future of hospital care in the United Kingdom, the private finance initiative and waiting list management, and has recently published a study of publicly funded research and development.

**John Appleby**

John Appleby is Chief Economist at the King's Fund. John has researched and published widely on many aspects of health service funding, rationing, resource allocation and performance. He previously worked as an economist with the NHS in Birmingham and London, and at the universities of Birmingham and East Anglia as Senior Lecturer in health economics. He is a visiting Professor at the Department of Economics at City University. John has recently completed an independent review of the health and social care system in Northern Ireland on behalf of the government.

# Acknowledgements

We would like to thank the following for their helpful comments on earlier drafts of this publication:

Seán Boyle, Senior Research Fellow, Health and Social Care, London School of Economics
Jennifer Dixon, Director, Health Policy, King's Fund
Chris Ham, Professor of Health Policy and Management, University of Birmingham
Mike Harley, Director, Inter-Authority Comparisons and Consultancy, Health Services
    Management Centre, University of Birmingham
John Yates, formerly Professor, Inter-Authority Comparisons and Consultancy, Health
    Services Management Centre, University of Birmingham

# Glossary

## BOOKING

For most of the life of the NHS patients have been put on to the waiting list and told subsequently when their appointment or operation will be. Booking requires that they are informed or choose when they will be seen or treated at the time of decision. The term 'partial booking' is used when a patient receives a firm date at some subsequent time a few weeks before the date of the operation.

Government statements about the booking programme have typically used airlines as the model they were aiming for. In one respect this is a curious comparison to make: although it is easy to make an airline reservation, airline booking systems are not always user-friendly because it is the norm to overbook. Nevertheless, planes normally do fly approximately when they are scheduled to. The difficulty facing a booking programme in an acute general hospital is that it cannot easily manage its emergency demand on a day-to-day basis, and hence it does not reliably know what its capacity to treat will be. Booking patients effectively ignores that uncertainty or assumes it will be dealt with in some other way.

## ELECTIVE CARE

In NHS statistics elective care comprises two types of admission for hospital treatment (including day cases): planned treatments, which are those carried out at prescribed intervals such as dialysis; and waiting list admissions, which are the focus of this paper.

## ELECTIVE CARE SYSTEM

*See* Annexe 1, p 61.

## PATIENT PATHWAY/PATIENT JOURNEY

These terms refer to the various stages through which a patient passes from initially seeking treatment through to post-operative care. The pathway/journey may set out the institutions a patient passes through as well as describing in detail all the processes involved in carrying out investigations and procedures within, for example, a single hospital (*see* Figure 3, p 7).

## PLANNED PROCEDURES

These include procedures that form a programme of care involving regular visits to hospital, as well as those carried out at an interval after an initial first operation, such as the removal of a second cataract at some point after the first.

## REMOVALS

Patients may be removed from waiting lists for a number of reasons: they may die, they may move to another part of the country, they may decide not to have the operation, or may not be well enough to have it and have no prospect of becoming so. In addition, patients may self-defer, when for some reason they are unable or unwilling to have an operation when they are offered one, or be suspended from the waiting list when they are medically unfit. Inappropriate use of suspensions has been one of the devices used by some managers to bring their data into line with government targets.

### TREATMENT CENTRES

There is no one model for a treatment centre. Typically their work is operationally or physically separate from the main hospital and they generally focus on a narrow range of procedures.

### WAITING TIMES

The total time a patient waits is not published in routine statistics. Hospital episode statistics do provide a 'start to finish' figure; however these include time when patients are suspended from the list (where this occurs) so on average they slightly overstate the true figure. Moreover, the data become available only nine months after the end of each year. Department of Health figures, now published monthly, are more up-to-date but they measure the length of time people have waited when the monthly census is taken. This means that patients 'in and out' within a month are not counted. According to Department of Health statisticians, the two sources of data tend to move in the same direction but they do diverge from year to year.

### WHOLE SYSTEMS APPROACH

What a 'whole system' is varies with context. However, the core idea is that a problem, for example shortage of capacity, should be investigated by considering not simply the scope for investing in more beds but also ways in which existing beds may be used more efficiently. This may require action on the part of the hospital itself but in another area of activity, such as improved admission procedures, or require measures within the community, such as the introduction of intermediate care beds to facilitate discharge.

# Abbreviations

A&E  accident and emergency

CABG  coronary artery bypass grafting

CHD  coronary heart disease

CT  computerised tomography

ENT  ear, nose and throat

HRG  health care resource group

MRI  magnetic resonance imaging

NPAT  National Patients' Access Team

PbR  Payment by Results

PCT  primary care trust

PTCA  percutaneous transluminal coronary angioplasty

# Summary

The need to wait for health care has been a feature of the NHS since its inception. This paper begins with a description of the task the Labour government faced when it came into power in 1997 and assesses the policy initiatives it has taken since then. It also looks at what the government should do next. The paper draws on previous studies by the King's Fund on waiting list policy and the ways in which individual trusts have responded to national targets.

When Labour came to power in 1997, total numbers waiting stood at 1.3 million – the highest since the NHS began in 1948. It pledged to reduce the number of people on English NHS waiting lists by 100,000 within its first term. That goal was achieved by 2000. The government went on to target waiting times, first by setting new maximum waits for outpatient consultations and inpatient treatment; second by setting a new target of 18 weeks covering the whole period from the initial GP consultations through to final treatment. This is to be achieved by 2008.

By the time of the 2005 election, substantial progress had been made in reducing the number of long waits. While average waiting times had not changed by much, waiting times for some operations such as cataract removals and some heart operations had fallen rapidly. So too had the total number of people waiting to be treated. By this time, however, some of the government's policies, particularly the greater use of privately run treatment centres, were only just starting to have an impact. The government therefore has reason to be confident that the 2008 target can be met.

Nevertheless challenges remain. Achievement of the target is threatened by a number of factors, such as financial pressures, unanticipated increases in demand, and staff shortages in critical areas. A number of steps can be taken to reduce these risks.

Even if the 18-week target is reached by 2008, the government needs to go on to define a new set of objectives that more accurately reflect the underlying NHS objective of providing equal access for equal need.

## Policy phases of the 'war on waiting'

The policies that the government has adopted, or currently has in place, in its 'war on waiting' fall into three phases: Phase 1 (1997–2000), Phase 2 (2000–2004) and Phase 3 (2005–2008 and beyond).

### Phase 1 (1997–2000)

During this phase Labour focused on reducing the number of people waiting rather than reducing the time of waiting, although it did undertake to maintain the Conservatives' existing Maximum Wait Guarantee of 18 months.

To achieve the target of 100,000 fewer patients waiting for treatment by the end of its first term, the government took action in two main areas:

■ Directing funds at specific initiatives: in 1998 the NHS Executive allocated £320 million to fund extra efforts to reduce waiting lists, followed by more money for specific initiatives. This money was made available on an *ad hoc* basis, and NHS managers were never in a position to make long-term plans for service improvements in the expectation that the finance would be available to implement them. Compared with later increases, the NHS budget only rose slightly in this phase.

■ Increasing operational and technical support: this was aimed at helping individual NHS providers meet their waiting times targets and disseminate the lessons learnt in individual trusts throughout the NHS. Specific initiatives included the National Patients' Action Team, which advised hospitals on how to improve practice, and collaboratives around specific areas of hospital work, which were designed to rapidly spread information about successful innovation.

These measures were backed by pressure on hospitals managers from ministers and the performance management system.

### ASSESSMENT OF PHASE 1

Waiting lists rose steadily after 1997, increasing the task the government had set itself. But by mid-1998 the first signs of a fall appeared and by early 2000 the government had achieved its target of reducing waiting lists 100,000 below the level it inherited.

By the end of Phase 1, however, the government had accepted that reducing the numbers of people waiting was an inappropriate objective given that what patients were most concerned about was how long they spent waiting.

New objectives were therefore required and a new set of policies.

## Phase 2 (2000–2004)

In March 2000 the Chancellor announced that the government would substantially increase NHS funding with the proviso that the NHS reformed. This was followed by publication of *The NHS Plan*, which, coupled with the increased funding, provided the government with an opportunity to develop new policies and modify the targets first set in 1997.

The new targets set for the NHS in this phase included:
■ abolishing waiting lists and replacing them with booking systems for patients
■ halving the maximum waiting time for routine outpatient appointments from more than six months to three months, and reducing the average time to five weeks
■ reducing the maximum wait for inpatient treatment from eighteen months to six, and the average time from three months to seven weeks.

These targets were accompanied by a wide-ranging set of policies to help transform the way that elective care was provided.

## INITIATIVES TO INCREASE SUPPLY

During this phase the government also introduced a number of ideas and programmes aimed at increasing supply within the health service:

- **Treatment centres** The main idea behind treatment centres was that they would have their work ring-fenced, that is, isolated from other hospital activities either through physical or operational separation. The private sector, in particular overseas providers, was invited to bid to run some treatment centre facilities, especially in areas where NHS performance was poor or there was an urgent need to increase capacity.

- **Day surgery** Sixty-six per cent of operations in 2000/01 were carried out on a day basis. The government aimed to increase this proportion to 75 per cent through promoting the wider use of day surgery.

- **Operational support initiatives** The NHS Modernisation Agency took over the existing operational support programmes and extended their scope. Before being drastically slimmed down, it published a vast amount of advice on how to achieve reductions in waiting times.

- **Speciality programmes** Ophthalmology and orthopaedics were two specialities with particularly long waiting lists. To help reduce these lists additional programmes were established in these specific areas.

- **Patient choice** Starting with a pilot scheme in London, the government gave patients facing long waits the right to go to another hospital. To enable the scheme to apply nationally, a new system known as Payment by Results (PBR) was introduced which directly linked a hospital's income to the amount of work it performed.

## DEMAND MANAGEMENT

Although the focus was on increasing supply, the government also supported the development of new services in community settings, such as GPs with special interests to reduce hospital referrals.

## IMPROVING THE WHOLE SYSTEM

To reduce pressure on hospitals the government set targets for increasing the overall number of hospital beds. It developed programmes that were designed to make better use of the existing bed stock by encouraging more rapid discharge of patients from both emergency and elective beds.

## SYSTEM MANAGEMENT

The government also introduced a star-rating system to provide a measure of trusts' overall performance in order to distribute a (relatively small) performance fund. However, the use of the star-rating system expanded to identify trusts in need of 'special measures' (for example, franchising of a senior management team) and to select potential candidates for foundation trust status. Five out of the nine 'key targets' of the star-rating system were related to waiting. The Department of Health's performance-management system meant that hospital management remained under strong pressure to meet waiting time targets.

**ASSESSMENT OF PHASE 2**

The targets for eliminating long waits were met during this phase but the numbers of people treated on the waiting list actually fell during this phase. Seemingly at odds with this, so did the numbers waiting. There were a variety of possible reasons for this:

■ The number of some procedures carried out declined sharply in line with an evidence-based approach, which identified some treatments, such as tonsillectomies, as being of low therapeutic value.

■ Some procedures were reclassified as planned operations or treated as diagnostic (neither planned operations nor diagnostic procedures are included in waiting lists).

■ There was a significant reduction in the number of people put onto the waiting list, which pointed to some degree of 'informal demand management'.

The measures introduced in this phase to improve capacity and overall system performance had little impact during this period. In particular, treatment centres ran with spare capacity, while private sector and overseas providers only made very modest contributions to reducing waiting lists.

Nonetheless, the government's policies set out in Phase 2 represented substantial progress compared with the previous phase. Overall, policy objectives were significantly improved by the introduction of targets set in terms of a progressive reduction in maximum waiting times. And for the first time in the history of the NHS, these objectives were set within a long-term framework, backed by a sustained increase in resources.

## Phase 3 (2005–2008 and beyond)

In 2004 the government announced a new target for the NHS: by 2008, no one should wait longer than 18 weeks from referral by a GP to hospital treatment. By setting a target that took into account the total time patients waited, the government acknowledged that waiting for diagnostic tests and their results, not previously counted in the statistics as 'waiting', was just as important as waiting at other stages of the patient journey.

The government felt that if this target could be achieved then waiting for elective care would cease to be the major concern facing the NHS. It could then tackle other priorities, in particular, increasing the quality of life of people with long-term chronic health conditions.

Although the 18-week target is a challenging one, the government has reasons to feel optimistic about the capacity of the NHS to reach it. Some of these include:

■ The total number of people waiting for treatment has continued to fall rapidly since 2004.

■ The extra capacity purchased in the private sector has begun to become available, and this will increase.

■ In early 2005 it agreed to £3 billion worth of contracts with the private sector to overcome shortfalls in diagnostic capacity.

If all the policies in place by the middle of 2005 work in line with government expectations, the NHS elective care system will shortly be transformed from the 'command economy' of the first two phases into a quasi-market economy. Hospital trusts will be put under unprecedented pressure from patients exercising choice (and taking the finance for their treatment elsewhere), other trusts offering quicker access and the private sector potentially removing business out of the NHS altogether.

However, there are some potential constraints that may affect the ability of the NHS to respond in the way the government hopes:

■ The financial climate is becoming less favourable than it was in the years between 2000 and 2005.

■ It will be increasingly difficult for the NHS to continue to make progress with reducing waiting because it has proved far easier to make rapid reductions in *maximum* waits rather than *average* waits. As long waits continue to be eliminated, improvements will have to be made for shorter waits, which involves reducing the waiting time for many more patients.

■ The government's estimates of the extra capacity required may prove to be wrong. There is a possibility that if waiting times reduce, demand will increase – for example, with more people moving from the private sector and GPs making more referrals.

■ There will probably continue to be shortages of key personnel (for example, in diagnostics and particularly radiology).

■ Trusts and patients may not respond to recent policy changes in the way the government expects. Payment by Results, for example, will be effective only if some trusts are able to expand and are prepared to accept the risks of doing so. Furthermore, it is uncertain how far patient choice will influence change.

### ASSESSMENT OF PHASE 3

The targets set during Phase 3 represent a further improvement over those developed for the previous two phases. The current 18-week target – which combines waiting at all stages of the patient journey – reflects the actual experience of patients better than the targets that have preceded it. It also reduces the potential for measured aspects of care to be improved at the expense of previously unrecorded factors such as diagnostic waits.

The policies in place to achieve the new target, particularly the expansion in diagnostic and treatment capacity, should result in further reductions in waiting times. The risks identified above may be reduced by suitable policies.

Nevertheless, if the 2008 target is met, that will not represent an end to wating.

## Meeting the 2008 target: what else needs to be done?

From Phase 1 to Phase 3 the government improved the way it expressed the waiting reduction targets it set for the NHS. Nevertheless, there remain a number of contentious questions that the government has yet to resolve if the objectives for access to elective care are to be properly framed. These include:

■ **Should there be a national target?** Setting targets has helped to achieve the changes in the NHS that the government has been pursuing. While the practice of setting targets should be retained, it may be that rigid adherence to them creates intolerable pressure in specific situations. This could be ameliorated by slightly relaxing the targets in certain circumstances.

- **Should the targets be more ambitious?** More timely treatment is the overall goal of targets to reduce waiting, however it is unclear whether the financial cost of eliminating waiting completely would be prohibitive.

- **Is the target too ambitious?** A single target does not reflect the complexities of the different treatment that people require. In some cases, such as cancer, the patient pathway should obviously be as short as possible. For other conditions, longer waits might be more acceptable, especially if patients know with certainty how long their wait will be.

- **Should targets be based on time alone?** The NHS is based on a principle of 'equal access for equal need'. On its own, a waiting time target cannot achieve this. Genuine equity of access requires a wide range of policies, and there needs to be more progress across other areas of policy-making to support this.

The policies now in place to support the target contain risks related to both demand and supply:

- **Demand side risks** Demand may rise more rapidly than has been assumed when the 18-week target was set, leading to insufficient capacity. Some form of demand management may therefore be required.

- **Supply side risks** These relate to the consequences of substantial increases in capacity and the workforce and systemic issues this will raise, especially around Payment by Results and the role of the private sector.

## Key recommendations

The government's determination to reduce waiting times in the English NHS has been rewarded with significant falls. To ensure that these achievements are sustained, the government needs to further develop:
- its objectives for waiting lists
- the policies that will achieve these objectives
- its understanding of the overall health system and, within that, what causes waiting.

### Objectives

The government should:
- give more emphasis to reducing differences in access levels between similar populations
- undertake more research to better understand variations in clinical priorities and treatment thresholds, as part of a more systematic programme of demand management
- assess what the overall benefits would be for patients, and the costs and benefits for the NHS, of setting even more challenging targets for the NHS beyond the current 18-week target
- monitor future patient choices and potentially use these as the basis for setting objectives for access to elective care; this would mean a shift from centrally imposed universal targets to ones that reflect the preferences of individuals.

## *Policies*

The government's present mix of policies are subject to a number of demand and supply side risks. To reduce these risks the government should:

■ carefully monitor the impact of Payment by Results and adjust this policy if it leads to a net reduction in the number of NHS operations, or to an increase in emergency admissions

■ pursue the agenda already set out for improving the supply of scarce skills (for example, in anaesthesia and radiology)

■ monitor whether the policies it has introduced to better manage long-term conditions lead to reduced hospital admissions and lower overall NHS costs

■ ensure the right balance between new capacity and better use of existing capacity, and between further ring-fencing of elective care and better management of elective and emergency flows within individual hospitals.

## *Understanding the system*

The government should:

■ improve monitoring frameworks and management systems nationally and locally

■ increase its understanding of the effect of new policies on the elective care system

■ improve the costing and financial control of the patient journey

■ make the model for health decision-making more explicit and, like the Treasury model of the economy, open for everyone to assess and use to make their own forecasts

■ ensure greater consistency between data about the elective care system so that it gives a reliable picture of how the overall health care system is working.

# Introduction

If there is one aspect of the patient experience of health care that the British NHS is known for, it is the need to wait. On the day it opened its doors in 1948, the NHS took on a waiting list of around half a million patients. Since then, numbers have risen and the waiting time for patients to see a specialist as an outpatient, or to be admitted to hospital, has increased.

For decades, patients and the public have been remarkably stoical about waiting. In part they no doubt see waiting as an inevitable consequence of a service that is free at the point of use. And yet, in numerous surveys over many years, the public has consistently listed waiting as the top problem with the NHS. In studies of the reasons why people choose to use private health care, long NHS waiting times – or at least the perception of the need to wait a long time – are also cited as important.

Over the last 30 years there have been numerous attempts to reduce both the total numbers of people waiting and waiting times. Some have been successful, at least for a time; others have failed. None has really got to grips with the reasons why waiting lists exist or has fully understood that tackling waiting times is not a one-off, isolated activity of little consequence to the rest of the health system.

When Labour came to power in 1997 it pledged to reduce the number of people waiting for hospital treatment. Three years later, with the publication of *The NHS Plan* (Department of Health 2000a), it committed the NHS to a sustained assault on waiting times and launched a wide range of policies designed to reduce these times.

Only recently, as waiting times have started to fall dramatically in England, can the full implications of what it has taken to achieve such historic reductions be appreciated. Reducing waiting times has not just been a case of throwing money at the NHS. It might be an exaggeration (though not by much) to suggest that cutting waiting times has been the main reason for all the big policy changes introduced over the last five years or so. It may also be an exaggeration (again, not by much) to suggest that the process of cutting waiting times has started to change attitudes within the NHS, including a renewed focus on the patient and their experience of the health care system.

Reducing waiting times has made those responsible for the NHS think more deeply about how the health system works as a whole, how elective care interacts with referral and emergency systems, and the way patients travel through the NHS from when their illness develops to their discharge from hospital. At the same time, reducing waiting times has been a critical test of the capacity of the NHS to change and of the government's policies towards it.

The successes of the last few years in England – the rest of the United Kingdom is another story – prompted a key statement in the government's follow up to *The NHS Plan* (Department of Health 2000a): *The NHS Improvement Plan* (Department of Health

2004a). This statement asserted that patients would be admitted for treatment within a maximum of 18 weeks from referral by their GP. By 2008 – the date set for achieving the target – waiting times will cease to be 'the main concern' for patients and the public (provided, of course, the target is met). This paper aims to assess whether the 18-week target is likely to be achieved, what the government should do to increase the chances of success and, if the target is achieved, what policies should be adopted subsequently to build on that success.

This paper begins with a brief description of the task the government faced when it came to office in 1997, drawing on previous studies by the King's Fund (for example, Harrison and New 2001) into waiting list policy at the national level in England. The main part of the paper assesses the policy initiatives the government has taken. In doing so, it draws on another King's Fund study (Appleby *et al* 2004), which examined the way individual trusts responded to the nationally set targets. The final section of the paper examines what the government should do to increase its chances of success, and what to do next if the 18-week target is achieved.

---

### WHY DO WAITING LISTS EXIST?

In his classic study of waiting lists in the English NHS, John Yates (1987) posed the simple question: why is Mrs X waiting so long for the operation she needs? The answer proved to be far from straightforward. Twenty years later, the answer remains equally complex. There are several competing or possibly complementary explanations.

**Theory 1**: The waiting list represents a backlog of work arising from a temporary surge in demand or temporary shortfall in supply. If this theory were correct then NHS spot-purchasing from the private sector or weekend working would solve the problem. One sure lesson from experience in the United Kingdom and elsewhere is that waiting lists cannot be dealt with in this way.

**Theory 2**: The NHS waiting list is a device used by NHS consultants for encouraging patients to be treated privately – by the same consultants. This theory, not surprisingly, is strongly rejected by NHS consultants, who point to the long hours they work and the limits on the number of operations they can do due to factors outside their control, such as access to operating theatre time. A more plausible version of this theory may be that, because the affluent can bypass NHS waiting lists, political pressure to deal with waiting lists has been relatively muted. The government – in public at least – has not espoused Theory 2, but it has been put forward vigorously by John Yates (1987) and Donald Light (2000).

**Theory 3**: The waiting list is a device for rationing demand in a cash-limited system. It would disappear if more resources were devoted to eliminating it but, for reasons of expenditure control, it may be necessary to ration access to care.

**Theory 4**: The waiting list exists because the system currently performs much below its potential; the list could be removed by better performance.

From 2000 onwards, the government has acted on the assumption that a combination of theories 3 and 4 are correct.

# 1 Fifty years of policy failure

**This section summarises the history of waiting lists in the NHS, including the record numbers of people waiting that Labour inherited when it came to power in 1997. It describes the failures of previous initiatives to reduce these waiting lists, but also highlights some of the pointers for what the policy goals should be for reducing waiting, and what may or may not work in attempting to meet these goals.**

The NHS inherited a waiting list for hospital treatment when it was established in 1948. Fifty years later, waiting lists were longer than they had ever been. This was not for want of attempts to reduce them. During those 50 years successive governments had taken a series of initiatives designed to reduce both the numbers of patients waiting and the time they waited.

In the 1980s and 1990s, for example, Conservative administrations had succeeded in reducing the numbers waiting for treatment for two or more years by introducing maximum waiting times as part of the Patient's Charter. In 1993 they introduced a measure of the time spent waiting to see a consultant and set a maximum here too. But these waits were still long by international standards. Some countries, including many on mainland Europe with broadly similar health care systems, had few or even no patients waiting as long as these maximum times.

However, by the end of their period of office in 1997, the Conservatives appeared to have given up hope of achieving further gains. The targeted funding under their Waiting Times Initiative started in 1986 and came to an end nearly a decade later. The Maximum Waiting Time Guarantee remained in place, but there was no sign that they intended to reduce the maximum waiting times any further. The planning guidance (NHS Executive 1996) issued to the NHS in the Conservatives' last full year of office simply reaffirmed that waits should be kept within the existing maximum of 26 weeks for the first outpatient appointment – with 90 per cent of patients to be seen within 13 weeks – and 18 months for inpatient treatment. The exceptions were coronary artery bypass grafting (CABG) and percutaneous transluminal coronary angioplasty (PTCA), where the limit was set at 12 months. Their final White Paper, *A Service with Ambitions* (Department of Health 1996) re-affirmed this position. Not surprisingly, numbers waiting continued to rise. As Figure 1 overleaf shows, many patients waited for over 12 months after they had been added to the waiting list.

The numbers waiting after the decision was made by a consultant to treat them was only part of the story. Patients also experienced long waits before they saw a hospital consultant (*see* Figure 2 overleaf); a significant number of patients were waiting over 26 weeks.

Many patients waited much longer than the figures suggest, particularly if they were referred for further investigations such as a computerised tomography (CT) or magnetic resonance imaging (MRI) scan. Waits for these procedures went unrecorded in national

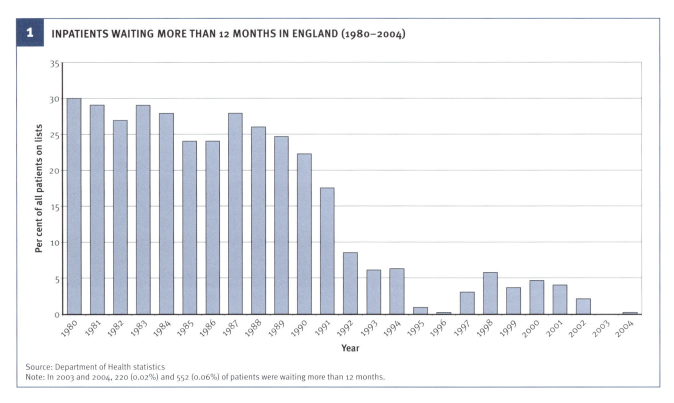

**1** INPATIENTS WAITING MORE THAN 12 MONTHS IN ENGLAND (1980–2004)

Source: Department of Health statistics
Note: In 2003 and 2004, 220 (0.02%) and 552 (0.06%) of patients were waiting more than 12 months.

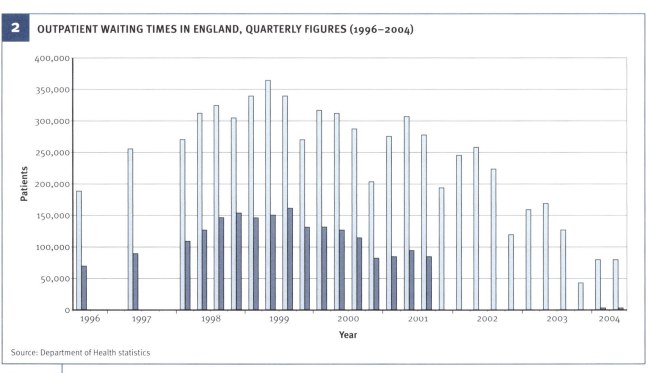

**2** OUTPATIENT WAITING TIMES IN ENGLAND, QUARTERLY FIGURES (1996–2004)

Source: Department of Health statistics

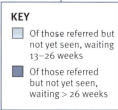

KEY

Of those referred but
not yet seen, waiting
13–26 weeks

Of those referred
but not yet seen,
waiting > 26 weeks

statistics. However, data collected in the early 1990s (Smith 1994) found that about one-sixth of the total delay experienced by patients arose while waiting between consultant lists.

For others, waiting was even more prolonged: some patients found that if they were unable to take up an offer of treatment their waiting time was 'reset' to zero. Hence, if their condition was not regarded as urgent, they went to the back of the queue.

Some patients did not even join the queue. Rates of treatment for common operations such as inguinal hernia repairs or more specialised procedures like CABGs varied more widely between different hospital trusts than could be explained by differences in needs (Clinical Standards Advisory Group 1993). Despite equity being central to the NHS, differences in access to elective care had never been systematically addressed. To what extent these arose from too much treatment in some areas and too little in others was unclear, but the implication of a number of studies (for example, Sanders *et al* 1989) was that some part of the variation was due to undertreatment. In other words, some patients did not gain access at all to the treatment they required.

The costs to patients of delayed access to care – or in extreme cases failure to gain access at all – had never been estimated. But a limited amount of research had shown that these costs were considerable, comprising long periods of pain or restricted activity, extra care costs, loss of earnings and, in some cases, loss of life (Harrison and New 2001; Hamilton *et al* 1996; Derrett *et al* 1999; Jonsdottir and Baldursdottir 1998). In addition, there were extra costs to the NHS arising from the treatment required during the waiting period to ameliorate the consequences of delay.

If the problem was so severe, why had it not been tackled more effectively? The answer is in part political. Although the Conservatives did tackle the longest waiting times, they feared that to set more ambitious targets would run the risk of failure with catastrophic electoral consequences. The Conservative Health Minister, Enoch Powell (1976, p 40), had warned in the 1960s that getting waiting lists down was an 'activity about as hopeful as filling a sieve'. It is therefore not surprising that the Waiting Times Initiative was allowed to lapse in the early 1990s once the longest waits had been eliminated.

But there is also a technical answer. None of the policy initiatives taken by the Conservatives or their predecessors had been based on an adequate account of the problem to be tackled. The Royal Commission on the NHS (1979) failed to provide one at the beginning of the 1980s, stating explicitly that it had no instant solutions to offer. The continuing rise in the numbers waiting during the Conservatives' time in office was evidence enough that they too had not found a solution.

Nevertheless, some lessons could be drawn from experience prior to 1997, in particular from the Conservatives' Waiting Times Initiative:

■ Waiting times rather than the length of waiting lists are what matter to patients.

■ Maximum waiting time limits can be effective in reducing the number of long waiters even if average waits do not change much.

■ Waits at different stages need to be monitored because improvements at one stage of the patient journey may be offset by delays at another.

- One-off cash injections targeted at waiting lists are unlikely to be effective unless other measures are taken. If waiting lists and times are to be reduced and kept low, appropriate policies must be put in place and sustained.

- Some form of technical support is required to help the worst performers in regards to waiting lists at hospital, speciality and individual consultant levels.

Most of these had been identified by the Health Committee (House of Commons Health Committee 1991) in the early 1990s, by other commentators (Yates 1987), and even earlier in respect of orthopaedics (Department of Health and Social Security 1981). Labour did not fully learn these lessons while in opposition. It came to office in 1997 with a clear commitment to reducing the *number* of people waiting for hospital treatment, but without a coherent strategy based on this earlier experience.

## Inheriting 50 years of failure: New Labour's war on waiting

From the time it came to power in 1997 through to the 2005 election, waiting lists – and subsequently the time patients had to wait – were never far from the top of the government's agenda. But both the precise objectives and the policies used to fight the 'war on waiting', as the government itself called it, changed during these eight years.

After its initial focus on the numbers waiting for treatment, the government went on to set new targets, first in *The NHS Plan* (Department of Health 2000a) and then again in *The NHS Improvement Plan* (Department of Health 2004a). As the targets changed, so did the policies – indeed, by the end of the period, policies had been adopted that had been explicitly rejected in 1997.

### *Assessing Labour's performance on waiting*

The remainder of this paper assesses Labour's record on waiting from 1997 to 2005 and examines the prospects of policy for the three years ahead to 2008, by which time, the government believes, waiting will have ceased to be of major concern.

The paper bases this assessment on three requirements for successful policy-making in this area:

- **What are the right objectives?** Should these be set in terms of numbers waiting? Or the maximum time any patient should wait? Or average waiting time? How should waiting be measured? Should objectives be set for specific conditions, with more demanding ones for those where time is critical? Should the same objectives apply to all parts of the country? How should objectives for improving access to hospital care be balanced against other health policy objectives?

- **What is the best mix of policies to achieve whatever objectives are set?** Is more capacity required and, if so, who should provide it? Or can the productivity of existing resources be raised sufficiently? If so, what policies are the most likely to succeed in producing the changes required to make them more productive: targets, incentives or new ways of working?

- **How will the elective care system develop in the absence of any attempt to change it and how will it respond to changes introduced with the aim of improving its performance?** What developments in medical technology might increase or reduce the scope or need for treatment? If waiting times fall will more patients seek care? How will NHS managers and clinicians react to attempts to change the way that treatment is provided? What will be the impact of other policies, for example emergency care, on the way that the elective care system operates?

The following three sections divide up Labour's 'war on waiting' into three phases, in line with the three sets of objectives it set for improving access to elective care. The emphasis in Phase 1 was on reducing the numbers waiting for treatment. In Phase 2, this switched to an emphasis on the time people spent waiting for an initial appointment with a hospital specialist and then subsequently for treatment. In Phase 3, concern widened to include *all* forms of waiting throughout the length of the patient journey, from initial consultation with a GP to final treatment (*see* Figure 3).

**3** A PATIENT'S JOURNEY (OR THE 'PATIENT PATHWAY') THROUGH THE HEALTH SYSTEM

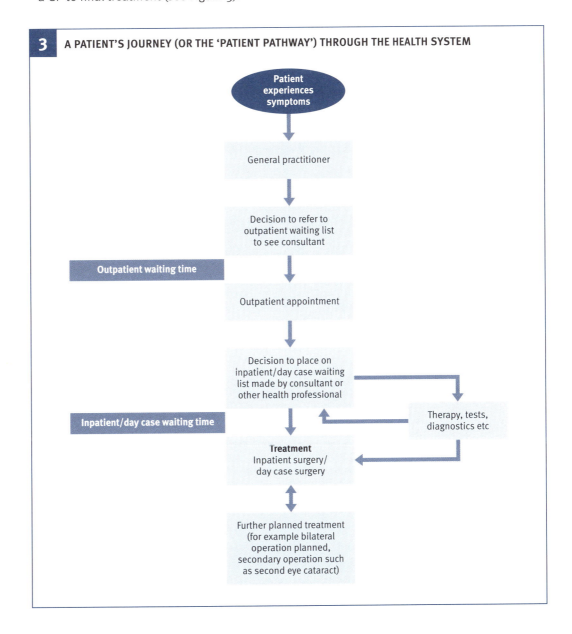

# 2 Phase 1 (1997–2000): Piecemeal policy-making

**This section summarises what Labour did to tackle waiting lists in its first term to 2000. It sets out the various initiatives and analyses their policy impact. It shows that, while some progress was made, by 2000 waiting times had not fallen and the number of waiting list operations carried out by the NHS had scarcely risen. The overall finding is that during this phase the underlying problems were not systematically addressed.**

The government came to office in 1997 with a commitment to reduce the number of people waiting by 100,000 below the level it inherited, within the life of its first Parliament. At that time, total numbers waiting stood at 1.3 million, the highest since the foundation of the NHS.

Despite the political importance of achieving the target little was done in 1997 to achieve it. Labour's first White Paper, *The New NHS* (Department of Health 1997), contained no proposals bearing directly on waiting lists. However, from 1998 onwards the government made it clear to the NHS that the target had to be met. The message was conveyed directly by the then Secretary of State Frank Dobson and his ministers to NHS Trust chairs and chief executives in a series of face-to-face meetings in early 1998. Chief executives and chairs of trusts were under no illusion as to the key indicator of their performance.

This pressure was maintained through the NHS performance management system. The planning guidance issued to the NHS for 1998/99 confirmed the government's commitment to the 100,000 figure and to maintaining the existing Maximum Wait Guarantee of 18 months, the target inherited from the Conservatives (NHS Executive 1997). It also required health authorities 'to ensure that the number of 12 month waits and outpatient performance are managed vigorously' (para 23), but did not set a specific target for either.

The government adopted two direct approaches to achieving these objectives: targeted injections of funds; and operational and technical support. It also used one indirect approach: the development of a booking system for outpatient appointments and hospital admissions, particularly for day cases.

## Targeted funding

During the first year of the government's first term, the NHS received only a modest increase in funding. However, in March 1998 the Chancellor announced an increase in the overall NHS budget. In the following month the NHS Executive said that £320 million of this would be allocated to fund additional efforts to reduce waiting lists, some of it in the form of 'rewards' for successful trusts (NHS Executive 1998a; Department of Health 1998a). Later that year, the national priorities guidance issued by the Department of Health (1998b) for the following two years stated that some of the extra resources would be ring-fenced into a Modernisation Fund, which was to be used to promote specific objectives including reductions in waiting lists. A series of cash injections followed: for example, in February 1999, £20 million was allocated for new operating theatres and surgical and diagnostic equipment, and in August 1999 a £30 million performance fund was set up to support reductions in waiting lists and times (Department of Health 1999a, 1999b).

It is not possible to establish exactly how these extra funds were used. Some paid for extra physical capacity, useful in the medium to long term, but much of it went on short-term measures such as overtime payments to clinical and other staff for weekend working.

Overall, around £737 million was committed through ad hoc injections of cash between 1998–99 and 2000–01 (National Audit Office 2001a). However, at no time during this period, or indeed subsequently, was an overall budget defined for elective care. As a consequence, NHS managers were never in a position to be confident about the availability of additional funds in the future and therefore could not make long-term plans for service improvements in the expectation that the finance would be available to implement them.

## Operational and technical support

During the Conservatives' drive in the 1980s to cut down waiting times the worst performing trusts received advice from outside experts (House of Commons Health Committee 1991). When the Waiting Times Initiative came to an end, central support of this kind virtually ceased. The Labour government initiated a number of approaches to help individual NHS providers meet their waiting times targets and disseminate the lessons learned in individual trusts throughout the NHS.

### National Patients' Access Team

In 1998 the government established the National Patients' Access Team (NPAT), which initially aimed to:

- help the NHS achieve sustainable reductions in waiting lists and waiting times
- invest in innovation through service redesign and quality improvement
- disseminate examples of excellence in practice.

To carry out these functions the team visited hospitals to advise on improvement, provided coaching in service redesign and helped to support the dissemination of successful examples of practice (*see* The work of the National Patients' Access Team overleaf).

### Whole systems approaches

Separately from the work of NPAT, the government came to recognise that the way in which the elective care system worked depended on what was going on elsewhere within hospitals and in the community at large. Winter crises in the late 1990s forced hospitals to cancel elective operations, which of course made it harder to reach the waiting list target. The 1998–99 planning guidance (NHS Executive 1997, para 28) stated that work should be carried out locally to 'increase understanding of the interplay between emergency admissions, elective care and finance'.

The whole systems approach (Waiting List Action Team 1999) recognised that all the main activities of an acute hospital are interrelated; hence, any policies directed at improving performance in one area should also consider their impact on other areas and

---

**THE WORK OF THE NATIONAL PATIENTS' ACCESS TEAM: AN EXAMPLE**

During 1999 the National Patients' Access Team (NPAT) made a number of hospital visits which resulted in a brief report, *Variations in Outpatient Performance*. This contained a number of recommendations about how to improve the management of outpatient clinics, including what it called a partial booking system.

In 2000 the NHS Executive published further results of this study called *A Step by Step Guide to Improving Outpatient Services*. In the same year the Department of Health (2000b) issued *Tackling Outpatient Waiting Times: A new approach*, which reported the results of a knowledge transfer programme between what were referred to as NHS top experts and people in 11 hospitals responsible for managing outpatients. Later, another tranche of hospitals was added to the programme.

The message of all these documents was essentially the same: there was enormous potential for improving outpatient services through redesign and reorganisation.

---

vice versa. In 1996 an emergency services action team had been established to help hospitals deal with winter crises. From 1999 onwards the Department of Health made a team, known at the time as WEST (Winter Emergency Services Team), available to trusts to help them plan their overall capacity, initially during the winter months and subsequently more generally. This, like NPAT, was later subsumed within the NHS Modernisation Agency.

## *The collaboratives*

The department also offered technical support through a series of collaborative projects. In 1999 the Cancer Collaborative – a national programme initially involving 51 projects in nine cancer networks – was established as part of the booked admissions programme (*see* Booked admissions opposite). Although originally expected to last only two years, it was expanded following the publication of *The NHS Plan* (Department of Health 2000a).

The Cancer Collaborative, as its name suggests, was a shared learning approach, with those in each network exchanging experience of how to redesign a patient's pathway and other means of service improvement. It also embodied a series of guidelines on the provision of cancer services covering the main cancers. Later, other collaborative projects were established for additional areas of hospital work.

The initial focus on cancer was attributable both to a separate government commitment to improving cancer care and to the way in which targets for cancer were set. Unlike the government's approach to elective care as a whole, targets for cancer were set in terms of maximum times in recognition of the need for rapid access to diagnosis and subsequent treatment. Initially, the policy focused on breast cancer but was then gradually extended to all forms of cancer.

A two-week target for the time between GP urgent referral and outpatient consultation was announced for breast cancer soon after Labour came to power; this was confirmed in the White Paper *The New NHS* (Department of Health 1997) issued a few months later. An audit of cancer patient waiting times was carried out in October 1997 which showed that about 70 per cent of patients had been seen within two weeks. The two-week target required that all patients should be seen within this time (Department of Health 1998c).

The government recognised that the demanding nature of the target required action across different areas. This included new investment and recruitment of extra staff as well as redesigning the patient pathway to eliminate waits that reflected poor working practices rather than shortage of capacity. The collaborative approach was designed to ensure that experience of successful innovation spread rapidly.

## Action On programmes

Another series of learning projects known as the Action On programmes was also aimed at developing and implementing new working methods. The Waiting List Action Team (1999, p 20) described its aim as being 'to demonstrate the improvements in patients' access to care that can be achieved through an integrated approach within health communities'. The means included:

- reviewing local access rates
- reviewing process and criteria for referral
- redesigning the patient's pathway
- using advanced surgical techniques
- enhancing staff roles and skills to support the redesigned process.

The Action On programmes initially focused on cataracts and went on to include other specialties with long waits such as ear, nose and throat, dermatology, urology and orthopaedics.

## Booked admissions

The National Booked Admissions Programme was launched in 1998 with 24 pilots running from October 1998 to 2000. Previously, most patients needing elective care were added to a waiting list and given only the broadest indication of when they would be treated. The programme was designed to remove this uncertainty by giving patients an admission date at the point when staff decided that treatment was necessary, or very soon after. As the then Minister for Health with responsibility for waiting lists and times, Lady Hayman, said (Department of Health 1999c, p 1):

> We expect to be able to book travel tickets and make hotel reservations in advance. In a modern NHS it should be as straightforward as this for GPs to book hospital appointments for their patients and consultants to book operation dates while their patients are with them in their outpatient clinics.

The booking programme did not bear directly on waiting times. However, the government expected that improvements in waiting times would result from the changes in procedures that were required for booking systems to be introduced effectively.

The initial emphasis was on day cases. The government thought this would be the easiest place to start since many hospitals already operated free-standing day units that were more or less isolated from the pressures of emergency admissions. In principle, and in contrast to surgical wards for inpatients, they could plan ahead with confidence that their capacity would not be commandeered at short notice to deal with emergency patients.

In April 1999 the programme was expanded. This included bringing in a large number of additional pilot sites, extending the programme specifically to cancer and taking five of the initial sites as the focus for more intensive work. The national Cancer Collaborative (*see* The collaboratives opposite) was established as part of this extension. Participating centres were encouraged to utilise what was termed the 'rapid cycle' technique, which involved piloting changes on a small number of patients and then extending the use of successful techniques.

## Policy impact

Waiting lists rose steadily after 1997, increasing the task the government had set itself. But by mid-1998 the first signs of a fall appeared (*see* Figure 4 below) and the then Secretary of State for Health, Frank Dobson, was able to announce that 'the supertanker had turned' (Department of Health 1998d). In the following year, the then Health Minister, John Denham, announced the Outpatient Performance Fund and was able to report a reduction of 200,000 on the previous year (Department of Health 1999b). By early 2000 the government had achieved its reduction target.

There was a less dramatic improvement in waiting times. The number of long waits started to come down so that, by the end of March 1998, no one was waiting more than 18 months for treatment and very few were waiting over 15 months or one year (*see* Figure 5 opposite). But average inpatient and day case waiting times for treatment showed little change (*see* Figure 6 opposite) and outpatient median waiting times actually rose (*see* Figure 7, p 14). The numbers waiting over 13 weeks for an outpatient appointment also rose (*see* Figure 8, p 14).

Most importantly, although the number of patients treated from the waiting list rose between 1997 and 1998–99, it subsequently declined (*see* Figure 9, p 15). Official figures continued to show a rise in the number of non-emergency patients treated, but this total included planned operations, which did not contribute to reducing waiting lists (and hence

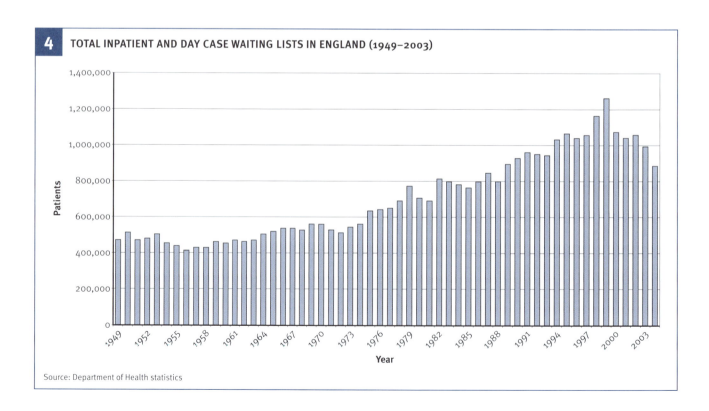

**4** TOTAL INPATIENT AND DAY CASE WAITING LISTS IN ENGLAND (1949–2003)

Source: Department of Health statistics

**5**  INPATIENTS WAITING MORE THAN 12 MONTHS AND MORE THAN 15 MONTHS IN ENGLAND (1995–2004)

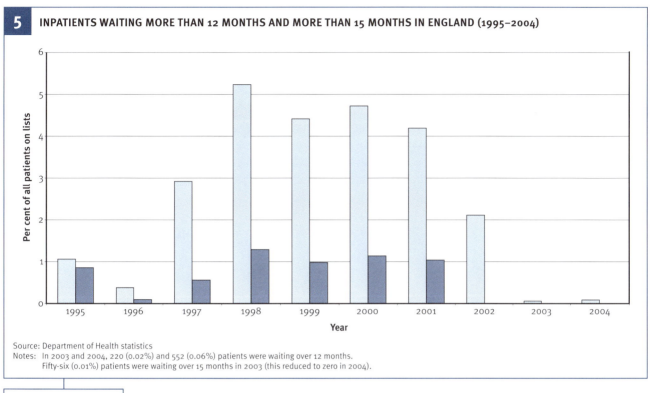

Source: Department of Health statistics
Notes:  In 2003 and 2004, 220 (0.02%) and 552 (0.06%) patients were waiting over 12 months.
Fifty-six (0.01%) patients were waiting over 15 months in 2003 (this reduced to zero in 2004).

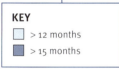

KEY
☐ > 12 months
■ > 15 months

**6**  MEAN AND MEDIAN INPATIENT WAITING TIMES IN ENGLAND, QUARTERLY FIGURES (1988–2003)

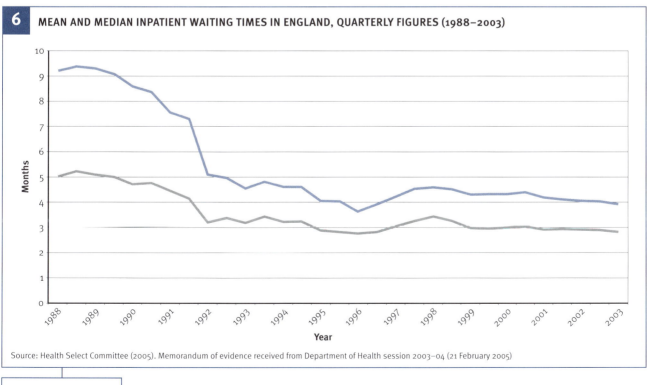

Source: Health Select Committee (2005). Memorandum of evidence received from Department of Health session 2003–04 (21 February 2005)

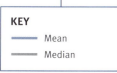

KEY
— Mean
— Median

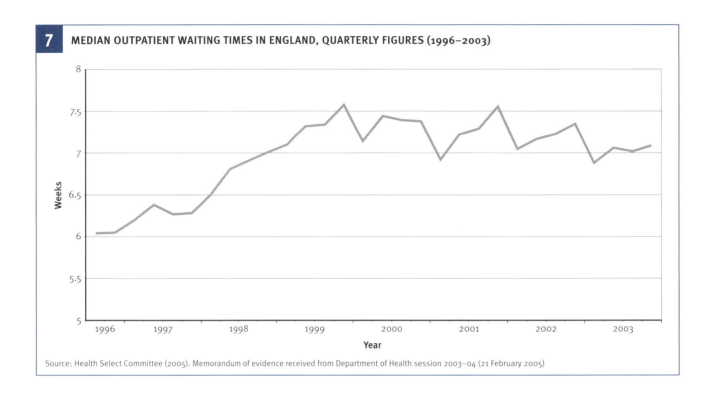

**7  MEDIAN OUTPATIENT WAITING TIMES IN ENGLAND, QUARTERLY FIGURES (1996–2003)**

Source: Health Select Committee (2005). Memorandum of evidence received from Department of Health session 2003–04 (21 February 2005)

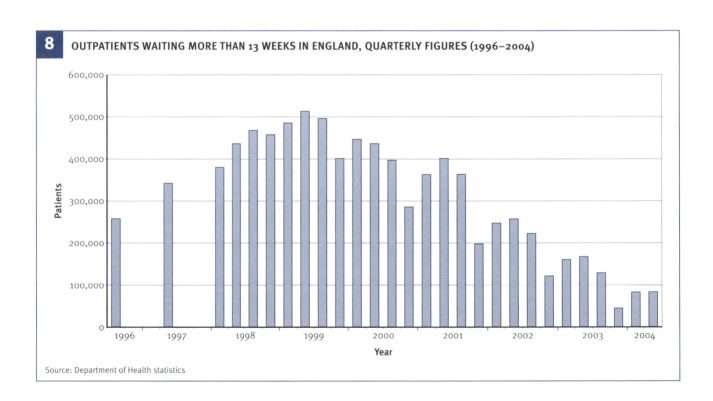

**8  OUTPATIENTS WAITING MORE THAN 13 WEEKS IN ENGLAND, QUARTERLY FIGURES (1996–2004)**

Source: Department of Health statistics

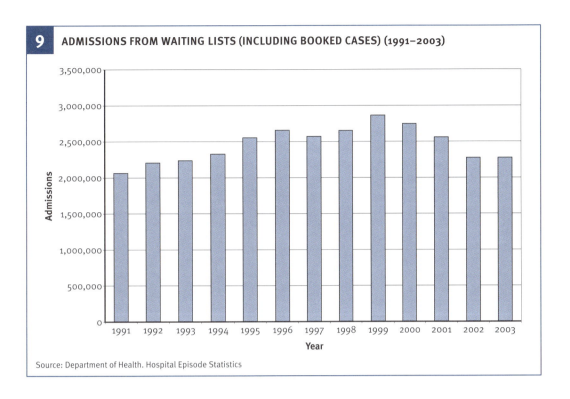

**9** | **ADMISSIONS FROM WAITING LISTS (INCLUDING BOOKED CASES) (1991–2003)**

Source: Department of Health. Hospital Episode Statistics

are not included in Figure 9). The rise in planned treatment masked, from 1998–99 onwards, the trend in waiting list admissions.

The waiting time target for breast cancer was nearly met, but at the price of longer delays for patients either further along the pathway or judged to be less urgent. A study of the time taken to receive treatment after referral since the introduction of the two-week limit between 1997 and 2000 found that the number being treated within five weeks of their hospital appointment had fallen from 84 to 80 per cent, and that the median waiting time for treatment had risen from 16 to 20 days (Robinson *et al* 2003). Another study found that patients judged to be less likely to have cancer were waiting longer after the target was brought in for those judged more likely to have cancer (Cant and Yu 2000).

These undesirable consequences appear to have resulted in part from a rise in the number of patients being referred to hospital for suspected cancer and the impact of the absolute deadline for seeing those judged to be urgent cases. Together they meant that hospital resources had been pulled towards the early part of the patient pathway from either later stages of treatment or from other hospital services.

In the pilot sites the proportion of patients booked rose and the number of people failing to attend treatment fell significantly (Department of Health 2000c). But there was little change in the overall percentage of admissions and consultant appointments that were fully booked, which had in any case been rising for some years (*see* Figure 10 overleaf).

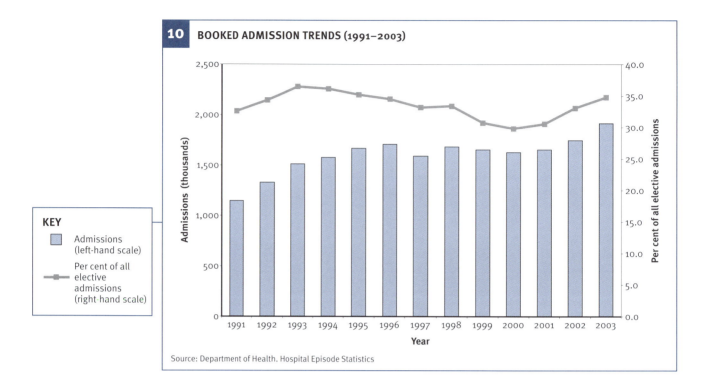

**10** BOOKED ADMISSION TRENDS (1991–2003)

KEY

Admissions (left-hand scale)

Per cent of all elective admissions (right-hand scale)

Source: Department of Health. Hospital Episode Statistics

## How were improvements in waiting lists and times achieved?

It is not possible to link the changes in waiting list performance to the cash injections made from 1998 onwards. In theory, allocations made to health authorities were linked to particular projects for improving the way the elective care system worked. But there was no overall budget for elective care at the national level, so there was no clear baseline against which to judge whether an appropriate increase in operations had occurred given the extra resources. In particular, it appears that no attempt was made to audit the series of cash injections to evaluate whether they were used in appropriate ways.

A subsequent study by the Audit Commission (2003a) indicated that the capacity to track hypothecated funding for this and any other purpose was still inadequate. Neither the government nor anyone else could say precisely how this funding was used and what it achieved.

There is only limited evidence of the impact of operational support during this phase. A report after the first 12 months of the Cancer Collaborative's operation (National Patients' Access Team 2001) stated that some projects halved the time from first contact to first treatment. But improvements such as these were unlikely to reflect experience across the NHS as a whole. Other collaboratives were not underway by mid-2000 and the Action On programmes had also not had time to make an impact.

However, Figure 11 opposite provides some clues as to how the waiting list target was achieved.

Numbers waiting can be reduced in three main ways: by treating more patients, by reducing the number of patients added to the list while keeping numbers treated the same, or by removing people from the list after they have been added to it. The National Audit Office (2001a) found that it was impossible, using national statistics, to make the various patient numbers associated with waiting lists balance without leaving some unexplained remainder. The big fall in waiting lists in the first half of 1999–2000 was mainly explained by an increase in the numbers admitted from the list, plus an increase in the number of patients removed from the waiting list. In contrast, the fall in waiting lists in the first half of 2000–01 was largely the result of an increase in the number of patients removed from the list; admissions from the list rose only fractionally. In other words, the reduction in numbers waiting during the second half of this phase arose mainly from better 'housekeeping' rather than a genuine improvement in access to care through growth in the numbers treated.

The changes recorded above were made against a background of sustained pressure from ministers and the NHS performance management system on hospitals to meet the waiting list and waiting time targets. No senior NHS manager could fail to be aware of what was required of them. This pressure did not determine what was done to meet the target, but it did ensure that all practical steps were taken to do so.

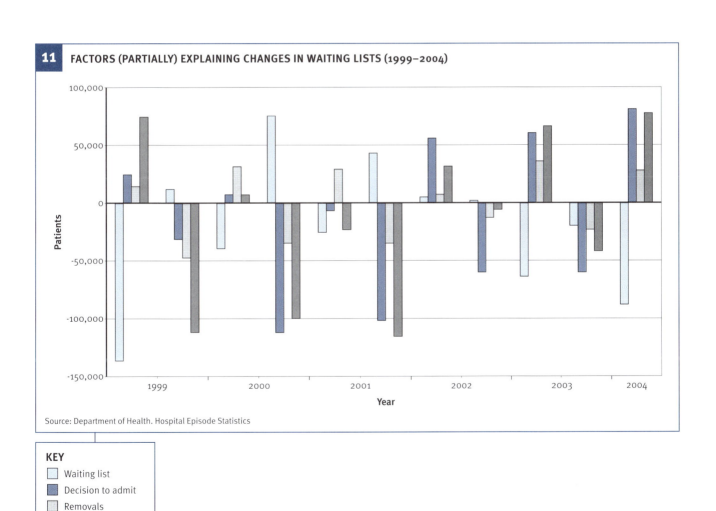

**11**  FACTORS (PARTIALLY) EXPLAINING CHANGES IN WAITING LISTS (1999–2004)

Source: Department of Health. Hospital Episode Statistics

KEY
- Waiting list
- Decision to admit
- Removals
- Admissions from list

## Overall assessment

Why was so little progress made during this period? There were four contributing factors. First, during Labour's initial three years the NHS budget rose only slightly (in real terms by around 1.5 per cent in 1997/98 and 2.5 per cent in 1998/99), and the use of dedicated cash injections did not guarantee that more would be spent on waiting list procedures. Although elective activity as a whole rose steadily, this was largely due to the planned component and had no impact on waiting lists or times (*see* Figure 12 below). However, it did absorb resources which, directly or indirectly, might have been used to carry out waiting list procedures.

Second, demand for elective care continued to rise. Referrals from GPs and other sources to outpatients increased (*see* Figure 13 opposite), as did referrals from other sources (for example, referrals from one consultant to another). The latter category of referral was not included in the waiting time statistics so no estimates of patient delays at this stage of the patient pathway are available.

Third, the productivity of the surgical workforce declined during this period. While the number of surgical consultants rose, their average number of operations fell (*see* Figure 14 opposite).

This trend – which was established before Labour came to power – reflected a number of factors including an increase in other claims on consultants' time (such as greater personal responsibilities in respect of emergency care and the training of juniors), more study leave as part of continuing professional development, and pressures on other hospital resources that reduced the efficiency of the surgical team and the effective use of theatres (Harley 2001; Galasko 2000; Robb 2002).

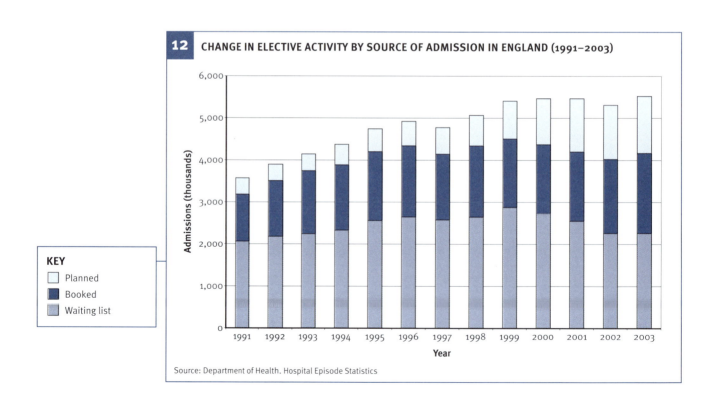

**KEY**
☐ Planned
■ Booked
▨ Waiting list

**12** **CHANGE IN ELECTIVE ACTIVITY BY SOURCE OF ADMISSION IN ENGLAND (1991–2003)**

Source: Department of Health. Hospital Episode Statistics

**13** REFERRALS FOR FIRST OUTPATIENT APPOINTMENT (1996–2003)

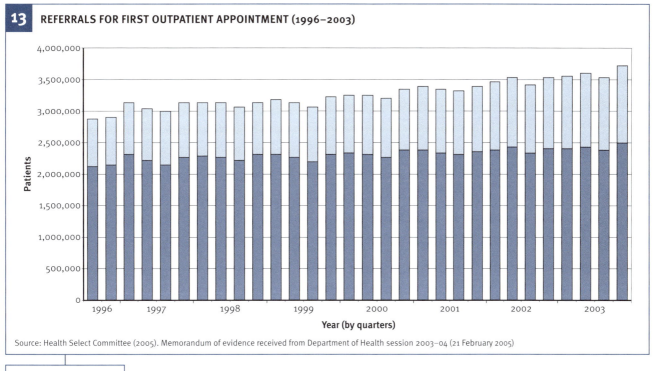

Source: Health Select Committee (2005). Memorandum of evidence received from Department of Health session 2003–04 (21 February 2005)

KEY

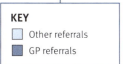

☐ Other referrals
■ GP referrals

**14** OPERATIONS PER HOSPITAL CONSULTANT (1992/93–1996/97 AND 1998/99–2003/04)

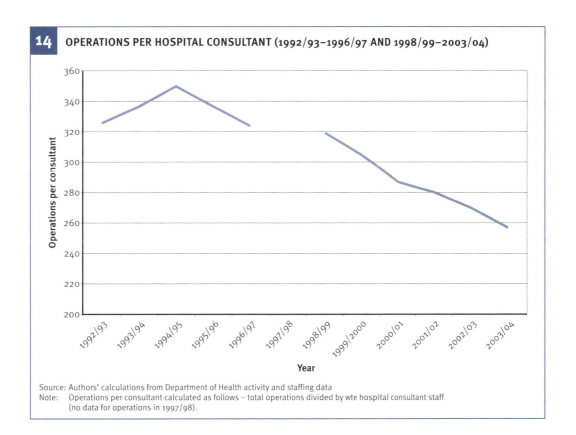

Source: Authors' calculations from Department of Health activity and staffing data

Note: Operations per consultant calculated as follows – total operations divided by wte hospital consultant staff (no data for operations in 1997/98).

Fourth, performance improvement in the absence of large increases in resources required changes in working methods. But the technical support initiatives outlined in this section did not begin to take effect until late in this first phase and affected only a small part of the total elective care system. The results, although worthwhile, were not large enough to have an impact on the national figures and even these gains proved hard to achieve.

The case of booking brings this out very clearly. There was already some experience of the problems involved in introducing a booking system, which demonstrated how difficult it would be to implement a national scheme; in light of this the government was right to introduce pilot schemes (Bensley *et al* 1997). In 1999 the Health Services Management Centre at the University of Birmingham was commissioned to evaluate the programme. A report issued later that year (Meredith *et al* 1999) acknowledged that booking systems represented an attempt to re-engineer or redesign working methods rather than simply to do more of the same. In other words, existing practices were not compatible with booking; this implied fundamental reform rather than a simple add-on to existing practices.

In their subsequent report (Kipping *et al* 2000) published in late 2000, by which time the programme had been extended to a large number of sites, the Birmingham researchers were able to report substantial progress in the pilot sites. But their report also reaffirmed that a large number of obstacles to extending booking existed, including insufficient capacity, rising demand, difficulties in recruitment, the impact of trust mergers, consultant resistance and misunderstanding among patients about the way the system worked.

Similarly, an evaluation of the first phase of the Cancer Collaborative found that respondents from a third of the pilot sites considered that the processes it involved were not well embedded in their organisation, even though the cancer teams participating in the pilots were likely to be the most progressive and receptive to change (Robert *et al* 2003).

In the light of these findings it is not surprising that NPAT's business plan for 2000–01 (National Patients' Access Team 1999) argued that, while piecemeal improvements could be made by short-term measures, service redesign was the key to effective modernisation of the NHS – but that this was not always feasible in the short term. The business plan also made it clear that there might be a shortfall in skills and the capacity to redesign services.

In brief, the policies adopted during 1997–2000 did not match up to the scale of the problem. On the positive side it could be argued that a good deal of learning had taken place through the various new technical programmes. But this learning had yet to be disseminated to all parts of the NHS. Moreover, it was based on only a limited amount of recent practical experience and analysis of redesigning the way services could be delivered.

## Summary of Phase 1

The measures the government took during Phase 1 were based on an inadequate understanding of the problem to be tackled.

First, policy objectives, apart from those for cancer, were set in terms of numbers waiting. From the outset the target of reducing waiting lists was criticised extensively (for example, see Hamblin *et al* 1997, 1998a, 1998b). But the government's commitment to it was so absolute – it was one of the so-called 'pledges to Britain' made during the election campaign – that it could not be modified during its first term in office. Why this particular target was chosen instead of, for example, planning reductions in the maximum waiting limits still operative within the framework of the Patient's Charter, is obscure. Ministers sometimes claimed that reducing numbers would also reduce the time spent waiting. But this may or may not be true, depending on the circumstances at the time. In fact, during the next policy phase, numbers waiting did start to fall dramatically, but average waiting times did not.

In the case of cancer, the government did adopt a time-based target. But it failed to consider the implications of this target and the extra workload it was likely to bring at other stages along the total pathway to cancer care. This affected all cancer patients, including those judged initially by their GP not to be urgent cases. Gains at the initial access stage for some were at the expense of longer delays later on in the process. In this case the right objective – speeding up access – was compromised by failure to understand how this particular part of the elective care system worked, and how it was likely to respond to the policies it was subjected to.

The same was true of the elective care system as a whole. The government used a series of cash injections rather than a sustained increase in funding. This was based implicitly rather than explicitly on the belief that, by carrying out more operations for a limited period of time, the list – which amounted in 1997 to about three months' work – could be substantially and permanently reduced. In other words, the number of patients waiting for treatment amounted to a backlog of work that could be 'mopped up' by a little extra effort such as extra theatre sessions, weekend working or spot purchases from the private sector. Hospitals used all these methods, often at high cost, to meet the waiting list target.

By defining the task as a catching up exercise, the backlog model seemed to remove the need for a strategy for fundamental change in the organisation of elective care services. It is not surprising that, instead of a well-argued and evidence-based strategy bearing on all aspects of elective care, the government took a series of separate financial initiatives rather than develop a sustained attack on the problem. Where it did take a longer view, by encouraging service redesign, too little was done in this phase to have a significant impact on the service as a whole.

In brief:

- The policy objective   a reduction in the numbers waiting – was inappropriate. It did not take into account directly what matters to patients, which is the time spent waiting for treatment.

- The successful achievement of the target for waiting numbers was due to pressure on hospitals to improve performance from ministers and the performance management system. The policy instruments were either short term or introduced too late to be effective during this phase.

- A foundation for policy-making – a correct view of how the elective care system worked – was lacking. In particular, a long-term framework was not established.

# 3

# Phase 2 (2000–2004): Towards a comprehensive approach

This section identifies the changes in targets and policies to reduce waiting times based on a significant rise in the NHS budget. It highlights that, by 2004, the government's more comprehensive approach to addressing the problem of waiting times was proving successful. The number of people waiting for long periods of time reduced dramatically and the total numbers on waiting lists also fell. However, average waiting times showed much less change. The section concludes by examining why further reductions would be difficult to achieve.

Against the background of only limited success described in the previous section, it is not surprising that in 2000 there was a sharp change of policy. This was made possible by a rise in the NHS budget.

In March 2000 the Chancellor announced substantial increases in NHS funding designed to bring spending on health in the United Kingdom to the (West) European average. *The NHS Plan* (Department of Health 2000a) which followed in July (also referred to here as the Plan) gave the government the opportunity to develop new policies and to modify the targets set in 1997, supported by the prospect of a sustained and substantial increase in funding.

The extra resources came with a proviso: that to 'earn' them, the NHS would have to reform. This was a mantra that the government applied across the public sector but with particular emphasis to the NHS. The stage was now set for a new campaign within the continuing 'war on waiting'.

## New targets

The first step was a change in targets. By the time *The NHS Plan* was being drawn up, the government had accepted that its original target was wrong, but because of its election commitment this target remained. Previous public consultation had established that, for the NHS, reducing waiting times was the main priority, after increases in the number of doctors and nurses. The Plan accordingly set targets in terms of maximum waiting times to be achieved by specific dates (see *The NHS Plan* waiting time targets opposite).

The form of these targets was significant because:
- they were set in terms of maximum access times, which all hospital trusts had to achieve
- the Plan envisaged a steady reduction in access times over a period of years – the reductions were to be achieved on a 'staged basis' (para 12.22), with the maximum waits being progressively reduced from 18 through 15, 12, 6 and 3 months.

For the first time, the notion of progressive and sustained improvement was introduced into policy-making for elective care.

---

### *THE NHS PLAN* WAITING TIME TARGETS

- *Waiting lists for hospital appointments and admission will be abolished and replaced with booking systems giving all patients a choice of a convenient time within a guaranteed maximum waiting time. As a first step towards this all hospitals will by April 2001 have booking systems in place covering two procedures within their major specialties.*

- *Assuming GP referrals remain broadly in line with the current trend in the growth of referrals, then the maximum waiting time for a routine outpatient appointment will be halved from over six months now to three months – urgent cases will continue to be treated much faster in accordance with clinical need. As a result of delivering this policy [we] would expect the average time for an outpatient appointment to fall to five weeks.*

- *The maximum wait for inpatient treatment will be cut from 18 months now to six months. Urgent cases will continue to be treated much faster in accordance with clinical need. As a result of delivering this policy we would expect the average time that patients have been waiting for inpatient treatment to fall from three months to seven weeks.*

Source: Department of Health 2000a, p 105

---

The additional financial resources becoming available to the NHS allowed the Plan to promise substantial increases in human and physical resources across the whole of the organisation. Despite the political salience of the waiting list target, there was no attempt to ring-fence or earmark these new resources for elective care or any other purpose. The practice of small targeted injections of cash for particular purposes continued. These were used, for example, to buy more cataract operations and to support the introduction of patient choice of hospital (*see* Choice, p 29).

Similarly, the planned increase in the number of hospital consultants did not specify either their specialties or how they would be deployed. Furthermore, by quoting numbers of staff rather than their actual availability to provide care and carry out operations, the Plan gave no indication of the effective increase in capacity that the nominal increase represented. The decline in surgical productivity and other relevant factors, such as the European Union Working Time Directive which reduced the hours worked by junior doctors, were not taken into account.

The Plan also did not specify how the targets were to be reached. It noted that their achievement depended on no sudden increases in GP referrals, but it did not specify what increases in activity were required or what other changes were necessary. In this sense it was not a plan at all but rather a set of aspirations. The detailed planning was to come with the publication of *Delivering the NHS Plan* two years later (Department of Health 2002a). Nevertheless, pursuit of the targets published in *The NHS Plan* led to a wide-ranging set of policies that aimed to transform the way in which elective care was provided.

## Increasing supply

*The NHS Plan* introduced a number of ideas and programmes aimed at increasing supply within the health service, including:

- treatment centres
- day surgeries
- operational support initiatives
- specialty programmes
- incentives for patients and staff
- a booking system called Choose and Book.

These are described in more detail below.

### *Treatment centres*

Despite its general lack of detail, the Plan did put forward a major initiative designed to increase the ability of the NHS to provide more operations from within its own resources or from the private sector. It proposed 'diagnostic and treatment centres', which have subsequently come to be known simply as treatment centres.

The key idea for treatment centres was that they would have their work ring-fenced, that is, isolated from other hospital activities either through physical or operational separation. This was not a new idea, even in the United Kingdom: for example, it had been tried in Wales in the early 1990s in individual hospitals (House of Commons Welsh Affairs Committee 1991). Typically, however, the pressure from emergency work proved too strong and the ring fencing broke down.

A similar objective was implicit in the widespread development of day surgery units in the second half of the 1990s. These were often physically separate from the main hospital. Even so, their resources were also sometimes poached for emergency use.

These pressures were intensified by changes in the way hospitals worked. Historically, surgical beds had been used as the 'safety valve' to deal with sudden increases in admissions. When hospital stays were longer there was usually a pool of patients whose discharge could be speeded up. Reduction in lengths of stay during the 1990s meant that most patients in hospital could not be discharged at short notice to free up a bed. In addition, the steady decline in the number of acute beds made it more difficult for surgical wards to be protected as most hospitals were operating at very high levels of bed utilisation with little slack on the medical and surgical wards. This meant that when a rapid increase in emergency admissions occurred, managers had little alternative but to cancel operations so as to make beds available.

In principle, ring fencing reduced if not eliminated the risk of cancelled operations. In the words of *The NHS Plan* (Department of Health 2000a, para 4.8), diagnostic and treatment centres would 'separate routine hospital surgery from hospital emergency work so they can concentrate on getting waiting times down'. At this stage the aim was to develop 20 centres by 2004; the number was expanded over the following years to 80 by the end of 2005.

The Plan also proposed that the NHS should make greater use of private sector facilities. In 1997 the government had turned its back on the private sector as far as provision of clinical care was concerned. But by 2000 the government was having to think again.

This change of heart was reflected in *For the Benefit of Patients* (Department of Health 2000d), a concordat that was foreshadowed in the Plan but published later in the year. It identified three areas for what the Plan termed 'co-operative working' (Department of Health 2000a, p 97); one of these was elective care that 'could take the form of NHS doctors and nurses using the operating theatres and facilities in private hospital or it could mean the NHS buying certain services'. At this stage the main emphasis was on any spare capacity that the private sector might have. It was left to individual health authorities or trusts to decide how to use whatever private sector facilities were locally available.

From 2002 onwards policy towards the private sector changed dramatically. In March 2002 strategic health authorities were asked to prepare capacity plans by June of that year – the first time such an exercise had been attempted across the NHS as a whole. They were required to provide both estimates of what the NHS could realistically do and their expected purchase of care from the private sector, including overseas sources.

The resulting assessments formed the basis for the conclusion that considerable additional capacity was required and this could only come from the private sector. At the time *The NHS Plan* was published, there was no indication of how large the private sector role might be. Initial estimates of the scale of its contribution came two years later: *Delivering the NHS Plan* (Department of Health 2002a) stated that up to 150,000 operations might be purchased from the private sector.

However, at this stage the private sector had only limited spare capacity. Moreover, there was a risk that any expansion of its role would reduce the capacity of the NHS since nearly all the private sector's surgical workforce was also employed within the NHS.

In June 2002 the Secretary of State issued a prospectus (Department of Health 2002b) outlining the approach that would be adopted in introducing new sources of supply; he also met with a number of overseas providers. The announcement emphasised that the aim of increasing the role of the private sector was to add to NHS capacity, not replace it, and that it represented a 'radically different' approach to that used in the past (Department of Health 2002c). This new approach included both importing clinical teams to be deployed in NHS hospitals and establishing physically separate units under private ownership.

In November 2002 the Department of Health issued a guidance note (Department of Health 2002c) on using overseas clinical teams. By this time a small number of hospitals had recruited staff, usually on a temporary basis and mainly from Germany and South Africa.

In December 2002 the department published *Growing Capacity: a new role for external healthcare providers in England* (2002d), setting out in detail the policies already announced in the prospectus. This argued that a new procurement programme was required because (p 1):

> *Improving patient experience... requires sustained increase in capacity, not just a short-term effort to clear waiting list backlogs. Sustaining lower waiting times while continuing to treat patients according to clinical need requires a permanent, structural increase in the volume of health care services delivered to patients.*

While the NHS could, it states, deliver some of this extra capacity, 'more... is needed if waiting times are to be reduced' (p 1). The programme was focused on cataracts and other ophthalmology procedures, orthopaedics and other day case work.

In contrast to the provisions of the concordat, the main elements of this programme were centrally run and the contracts for operations negotiated between the Department of Health and the would-be operators. In principle, the new treatment centres were to be established where current NHS performance was poor and the need for capacity greatest.

The commissioning process was open; it was advertised in the *Official Journal of the European Union* (known as the European Journal) in line with other public sector procurements. Although domestic private sector providers such as BUPA were allowed to tender, the process made it clear that overseas bids were particularly welcome.

In setting out what it was looking for from the new centres, the department emphasised three factors: innovation, productivity and speed. The latter was critical (p 1):

> ... *because the 2005 targets are the latest dates that the Department has got to have...* *permanent increase in capacity: the sooner the NHS can get this capacity on stream,* *the better we shall be serving patients.*

A key risk with expanding the private sector role was that new entrants would poach NHS staff. Those bidding therefore had to offer assurances that they would use resources not otherwise available to the NHS. In practice this meant that they should not employ anyone who had recently worked within the NHS (that is, within the last six months), but it did not wholly prohibit the employment of former staff who might otherwise have returned to work in the NHS.

In 2003 it was announced that the new centres would provide 250,000 operations a year – about 5 per cent of the then current level (Department of Health 2003a). Because most new private centres required new buildings it was not until early 2004 that this programme started to come to fruition when two mobile surgical units began operating.

Another less important initiative was use of overseas providers in their own countries. In fact, this policy could not properly be ascribed to the government at all. Its origins lay in the European Union. A small number of non-British patients brought successful cases before the European Court claiming that they were suffering undue delay in their own countries and had a right to be treated elsewhere and have this paid for by their own health insurers. After some delay the Secretary of State decided to endorse this policy for the United Kingdom in *Delivering the NHS Plan* (Department of Health 2002a). Subsequently, a number of health authorities, principally in southern England, started to send patients to France and Germany.

## Day surgery

There had been attempts to raise the proportion of surgery carried out on a day basis since the early 1990s. In 1990 the Audit Commission published a report that identified the scope for greater use of day surgery for 25 procedures (Audit Commission 1990). The Department of Health subsequently established a task force to promote wider use of day surgery.

The NHS Plan proposed that 75 per cent of all surgery should be carried out on a day basis. Data for 2000–01 show that 66 per cent of procedures were day surgery, not allowing for a large number of minor procedures carried out by GPs or in hospital outpatients, which are not counted as waiting list cases.

In 2001 the Audit Commission produced a further report which found that day surgery units were not being used to their full capacity. It estimated that an extra 120,000 operations could be carried out if they were (Audit Commission 2001). This estimate covered only the 25 procedures it had selected in its 1990 report as suitable for day surgery.

During 2002 a number of steps were taken to raise the numbers treated on a day basis. In August the Health Minister John Hutton announced (Department of Health 2002e) that £68 million would be made available over two years to expand day case surgery. At the same time the department published new operational guidance that proposed a number of additional surgical procedures as being suitable for day surgery (Department of Health 2002f). The guidance noted that previous work by the Audit Commission and the British Association of Day Surgery had found a number of obstacles to the effective use of day surgery units including:

- inappropriate selection of patients
- poor management of the flow of work
- clinicians' preference for inpatient surgery
- problems with mixing day and inpatient cases
- failure to recognise day surgery as a priority.

These were familiar enough problems – similar obstacles had held up the development of day surgery in the 1990s when the first centrally directed steps to promote it were taken. Indeed, the 2002 guidance (Department of Health 2002f, para 1.10) notes that its proposals mirror those of the Day Surgery Task Force published in 1993, however 'few have been implemented'.

## Operational support initiatives

*The NHS Plan* announced the establishment of an NHS Modernisation Agency (Department of Health 2000a, para 6.15) to 'help local clinicians and managers redesign local services around the needs and convenience of patients'. The new agency brought together the streams of work already mentioned – the National Patients' Access Team and the collaboratives in particular – as well as other functions. It was specifically charged with implementing more Action On projects in orthopaedics, dermatology and ear, nose and throat, extending the cancer collaboratives to every cancer service in the country, establishing similar programmes to cut delays in heart treatment and accident and emergency departments, and extending the booking programme.

The NHS Modernisation Agency was substantially wound up in 2004 as part of the quango cull within the health sector. But during the four years of its existence it published a vast amount of advice on how to reduce waiting times as well as carrying out a large number of consultancy assignments in individual hospitals and organising seminars to spread best practice.

Much of this advice was summed up in what was described as 'the definitive guide to modernisation' (Department of Health 2004b). The guide – *10 High Impact Changes for Service Improvement and Delivery* (NHS Modernisation Agency 2004a) – summarises what the agency learned. If these changes were implemented, the paper claimed, waiting lists would be virtually eliminated. They included:

- treating day surgery as the norm
- increasing patient flows by improving access to diagnostic tests
- reducing the number of queues (that is, pooling waiting lists) that bear directly on the execution of elective care.

The other proposed changes promised improved efficiency in other parts of acute hospitals and the wider NHS.

**TEN 'HIGH IMPACT CHANGES' FROM THE NHS MODERNISATION AGENCY**

Drawing on learning from its work, the NHS Modernisation Agency identified 10 high impact changes that organisations in health and social care could adopt to make significant, measurable improvements in the way they deliver care:

1. treat day surgery as the norm for elective surgery
2. improve access to key diagnostic tests
3. manage variation in patient discharge
4. manage variation in patient admission
5. avoid unnecessary follow-ups
6. increase the reliability of performing therapeutic interventions through a Care Bundle Approach
7. apply a systematic approach to care for people with long-term conditions
8. improve patient access by reducing the number of queues
9. optimise patient flow using process templates
10. redesign and extend roles.

The Agency claimed that if the principles were adopted systematically by the whole NHS:
- the experience of patients would be greatly enhanced by more appropriate and timely care
- hundreds of thousands of clinician hours, hospital bed days and appointments in primary and secondary care would be saved
- clinical quality and clinical outcomes would be tangibly improved
- it would be easier to attract and retain staff and there would be more enjoyment and pride at work.

Source: NHS Modernisation Agency 2004a

As in Phase 1 (between 1997 and 2000), a number of trusts devised improvement schemes of their own (Cocker and Elliot 2003; Burrows and Norris 2004). Some of these were publicised throughout the NHS within what was known as the Beacon scheme. A number of Beacon sites introduced innovations designed to improve access to elective care, details of which were made available throughout the NHS (NHS Modernisation Agency, various years).

## Specialty programmes

Two specialties with long waiting lists – ophthalmology and orthopaedics – were targeted for special attention. Ophthalmology was involved in one of the early Action On projects. In 2000, local health economists were asked to review their local services in the light of the report resulting from the Action On Cataracts initiative. In the same year £20 million was allocated from the Modernisation Fund for eye services to improve the patient pathway and to support a 50 per cent increase in cataract operations by 2003 (Department of Health 2000e, 2000f). The government allocated £56 million – later increased to £73 million – to reducing waits for treatment to under three months by December 2004 (Department of Health 2003b). Part of the NHS and private treatment centre programme was devoted to expanding capacity to carry out these operations.

Orthopaedics was recognised as presenting the greatest challenge for achieving waiting time targets. It too had been one of the Action On projects as well as a collaborative. A report based on this experience was published in 2002 with the aim of helping 'those involved in the provision of orthopaedic services to review their procedures in light of the wealth of experience gained by both the collaborative and Action On Orthopaedics' (Department of Health 2002g, executive summary).

However, by that time it was clear to the government that a more determined effort was required in this speciality. An unpublished report prepared during 2003 set out an integrated orthopaedics strategy aimed at the 40 trusts least likely to meet the six-month target by the end of 2005. Subsequently, the National Orthopaedic Project was established in early 2004. It was designed to focus the attention of local purchasers and providers on orthopaedics, to provide more support to the trusts least likely to achieve the six month target and to ensure that other elements of policy, including Payment by Results (PbR) and choice, supported progress in orthopaedics.

## *Improving incentives*

In the first policy phase the Department of Health exerted pressure on the NHS through the targets it set and the performance management system operated by regional offices and, later, strategic health authorities.

During Phase 2, pressure from the centre – that is, the Department of Health and the Prime Minister's Office – did not relent. But gradually an alternative approach to improving performance emerged based on the creation of financial incentives for both organisations and individual staff.

### CHOICE

In a speech to the New Health Network in 2002 the then Secretary of State for Health, Alan Milburn, combined the various policy streams set out in this section into a new vision of the NHS (Milburn 2002, p 4):

> *The balance of power has to shift decisively in favour of the patient. So now most fundamentally of all, our reforms will give patients a greater choice over services.*

There is little doubt that the initial reason for introducing choice was to achieve a reduction in the number of people waiting for six months or more. In December 2001 the Department of Health (2001a) had already published *Extending Choice for Patients*, which opened the way for choice of place of treatment. It stated that (p 2):

> *By 2005 all patients and their GPs will be able to book hospital appointments at both a time and a place that is convenient to the patient. Patients and their doctors will be able to consider a range of options. This might include the local NHS hospital, NHS hospitals or diagnostic and treatment centres elsewhere, private hospitals, private diagnostic and treatment centres, or even hospitals overseas... The point is by then, at the point of referral, the patient will be able to choose the hospital and the waiting time that is convenient for them.*

The policy was confirmed in *Delivering the NHS Plan* (Department of Health 2002a) in which the government announced that patients generally would be offered a choice of where they would be treated. In its words (para 5.4), 'Hospitals will no longer choose patients. Patients will choose hospitals.'

Initially, choice of place of treatment was introduced on a pilot basis for heart patients. In March 2002 the Secretary of State announced a £100 million fund to pay for more heart operations; hospitals were invited to bid to provide them (Department of Health 2002h). Beginning in July 2002, all patients who had waited six months were offered the choice of treatment at another hospital if waiting times were shorter there. In effect this meant that individual hospital waiting lists were merged into one. In October 2002 the Choice programme was extended to cataract surgery within London (Department of Health 2002i). Further funds were allocated to areas with high rates of heart disease and the maximum wait for heart surgery reduced to three months.

In February 2003 the Secretary of State, in a speech to chief executives (Department of Health 2003c), announced the extension of the heart scheme to other specialties. In London the programme was extended from mid-2003 to cover orthopaedics, ENT, urology, gynaecology, plastic surgery, oral surgery and general surgery. It was also extended in other parts of the country: for example, West Yorkshire, Greater Manchester and parts of southern England. It was subsequently announced (Department of Health 2003d) that from the middle of 2004 all patients would have the choice of at least one other hospital and, from December 2005, a choice of four to five providers (including a private one) at the time they are referred by their GP.

It is worth noting that while 'choice at the point of referral' implies a choice of hospital for inpatient care, it is really a choice about outpatient department. Most patients visiting an outpatient department do not then go on to be referred into hospital (via a waiting list). Quite how patients who do need hospital care make their choice of hospital was then, and remains, unclear.

## PAYMENT BY RESULTS

In its initial stages the Choice programme was financed out of central funds. But if patients were to be offered choice in this way a financial reform was required so that money followed the patient to the chosen hospital. As *Delivering the NHS Plan* (Department of Health 2002a, para 5.7) put it:

> *Those hospitals that have capacity... will earn more resources as the money follows the choice made by the patient. This is a sensible way of identifying and using spare capacity and... providing new incentives for hospitals to treat more patients more quickly...*

The emphasis on spare capacity was odd given that no hospital in the NHS at that time could be said to have any. More significant was the reference to 'new incentives': the introduction of PbR meant that the more work a hospital performed, the higher its income would be. Provided it was paid enough to cover its costs it would have an incentive to expand its capacity to treat patients. Although the government did not like to be reminded of this, PbR was in effect a reintroduction of the internal market that the Conservatives had established in the early 1990s and which Labour rejected when it came to power. However, a critical difference was that, while the Conservatives' market was confined to the NHS, Labour's comprised the private sector. This involvement of the private sector was set to expand rapidly.

The new PbR system started to come into effect on a partial basis in April 2003. The tariff priced all hospital activity, broken down into health care resource groups (HRGs). The key characteristic of the system is that, unlike the practice in other countries using similar systems, prices are fixed, currently on the basis of the national (English) average HRG cost. The choice of tariff is up to the Department of Health and ministers.

The system is intended to have two main effects: first, to enable patients to access hospitals with shorter waiting times or a perceived or actual higher quality of care than their local hospital; and second, to put pressure on hospitals to improve their performance.

The pressure comes from two main sources: through the loss of income if patients move to another hospital and through the impact of the fixed tariff. About half of all acute trusts had cost levels above the tariff level when it was announced and needed to cut their costs if they were to survive financially.

For the most part the government's aim of introducing incentives focused on whole trusts. However, in 2004 the Department of Health announced its intention to pilot a form of PbR applied at the local level, the aim of which was to provide incentives to individual surgeons (Department of Health 2004c). A report from the consultants Serco (Serco Health 2004) found that 32 pilot schemes had been established using a variety of incentives and covering some 8,000 inpatient and 6,000 outpatient episodes. The number of pilots was subsequently increased.

### Choose and Book

The potential of the booked admissions programme for encouraging reform of the way in which elective care was delivered was explicitly acknowledged in *The NHS Plan* (Department of Health 2000a, p 104), which stated that it 'acts as a driver for fundamental reform… it is part and parcel of the wider and more radical process of redesigning services round the patient, cutting out unnecessary stages of treatment, using staff more flexibly and reducing delays.'

The Plan goes on (p 104):

> *Booking appointments forces hospitals to organise their clinic slots and theatre sessions more productively. It also brings a dramatic reduction in the number of cancelled appointments and the occasions when patients just do not turn up.*

The Plan stated that by the end of 2005 waiting lists would be abolished and replaced with booking systems. In September 2000 the Secretary of State announced that, by March 2001, every acute hospital trust would be offering some booked appointments and, by March 2002, 43 hospitals would be offering them to all day case patients (Department of Health 2000g). The government allocated £40 million to help meet these targets.

From April 2001 onwards, booking systems spread from the pilot sites to all parts of the NHS under the programme Moving to Mainstream (Department of Health 2001b). The programme was intended to lead to 100 per cent booking of day cases by March 2004 and a significant (later defined as two-thirds) level for inpatient admissions.

While it was hoped that booking would help to reform the provision of care, the government also saw it as contributing to its wider objectives of making access to the NHS more convenient and making it easier for patients to choose where they would be treated. By 2004 the combined programme came to be known as Choose and Book.

## Demand management

The policies reviewed so far were all focused on the supply of care. The demand for care was almost entirely neglected. However, the government did support a number of developments designed to switch activity away from hospitals. *The NHS Plan* stated that by 2004 there would be some 1,000 specialist GPs who could take referrals from other GPs and carry out a wider range of diagnostic and minor surgical procedures. The idea was that this would reduce the pressure on hospitals. In 2003 the Department of Health also envisaged an expansion of nursing roles in community settings to reduce the need for hospital-based expertise (Department of Health 2003e).

The new GP contract finally negotiated in 2003 provided for so-called 'enhanced services' – in essence services that might otherwise be provided in hospitals. This opened the way for more activities to move from hospital to community settings.

According to the *Chief Executive's Report to the NHS* (Department of Health 2004d), around three-quarters of a million procedures were being carried out in community settings that might otherwise have been performed in hospitals. Most of these were not on the waiting list for treatment, but to the extent that hospital resources were released by transfer of these activities there may have been some benefit to waiting time policies.

In some localities steps were taken to manage demand for hospital services by, for example, limiting the number of referrals each general practice could make (Kipping *et al* 2002); these examples were rare. There was also evidence that hospital resources were being poorly used. The National Audit Office (2001a) found that, in general, consultants considered a high proportion of referrals – sometimes as high as 80 per cent – were inappropriate, despite the fact that some 850 referral protocols had been developed by then. This suggests that there was considerable potential for improving the referral process. No targets were set nationally for doing this, although a number of schemes were introduced by primary care trusts (PCTs) at a local level to reduce referrals.

## Improving the whole system

During Phase 1 the government had acknowledged that the way the elective care system worked depended on what was going on elsewhere in the health care system, particularly the workload imposed on hospitals by the requirements of emergency care. As noted already, the introduction of treatment centres was justified by the 'insulation' they offered from the pressures of emergency admission. A number of other policies were introduced (Department of Health 2000h) to improve the management of patients in ways that reduced the overall emergency workload, either in terms of the number admitted or the length of time they spent in hospital.

Another way of reducing the pressure on elective beds was to increase overall hospital capacity. Following the National Bed Inquiry (Department of Health 2000i), the government decided that the downward trend in hospital bed numbers should be reversed. The NHS Plan stated that the number of acute beds, including intensive care, would be increased. In particular, the Plan promised 7,000 extra NHS beds (2,100 of which would be in general and acute wards), 5,000 extra intermediate care beds, 1,700 extra non-residential intermediate care beds and a 30 per cent increase in adult critical care beds.

The government also aimed to make better use of the existing bed stock by encouraging more rapid discharge of patients from both emergency and elective beds. The problem of bed-blocking was an old one, which had frustrated earlier attempts to solve it. In 2002 the Department of Health (2002j) made the first of a series of allocations to increase the number of intermediate care beds to which patients could be discharged before going home. In 2003 the government decided on a new and more radical approach: it adopted a scheme that had been operating in Sweden whereby the cost of keeping a patient after they were judged fit for discharge fell on the local authority responsible for not making arrangements for their discharge in time. This provided a clear incentive to improve liaison between hospitals and local authority social service departments over discharge arrangements, and to put in place facilities such as intermediate care beds where patients could be discharged before they were ready to go home.

### System management

During Phase 1 the waiting list and cancer waiting time targets effectively drove performance. The political pressure to attain the new set of targets set out in *The NHS Plan* intensified: the Department of Health itself came under pressure from the Prime Minister's Office, where a delivery unit was established to monitor each department's performance against the range of targets they were trying to achieve.

The existing performance management process was also strengthened with the introduction of the star rating system. This was originally designed to provide a summary measure of trusts' overall performance in order to distribute a (relatively small) performance fund. However, the use of the star rating system expanded to identify trusts in need of 'special measures' (for example, franchising of a senior management team) and to select potential candidates for Foundation Trust status. Five out of the nine 'key targets' of the star rating system were related to waiting.

As a result, trusts were subject to the continuous but unpublicised pressure exerted by Department of Health officials, as well as pressure from their peers, local media and the public because of the very public process of having their performance measured and the results published.

## Policy impact

By mid-2004 the overall waiting list was falling rapidly. While this was no longer formally a target it was nevertheless interpreted by the government as a sign of success. Elimination of long waits in line with the Plan target for April 2004 had also been achieved (*see* Figures 15 and 16 overleaf). The target for day case booking had nearly been met although the majority of patients were still being offered only 'partial booking'. The proportion of full booking had failed to rise.

At service level the main targets had also been met. The three year progress report on cancer (Department of Health 2004e) found that the access time targets set for 2000, 2001 and 2002 had been met.

The 2004 progress report on the National Service Framework for Coronary Heart Disease (Department of Health 2004f) indicated that no one was waiting over nine months for an operation. Some of this decline had been achieved by increasing the number of operations. But service redesign had also made a contribution (p 34): 'Initial data from the CHD collaborative... has shown that redesign of echocardiography services reduces waiting times for inpatients from a median of 5.25 days to a median of 1.125 days'.

Other data suggested that performance had not markedly improved. Average waits for most procedures fell slowly with the marked exception of cataracts and coronary artery

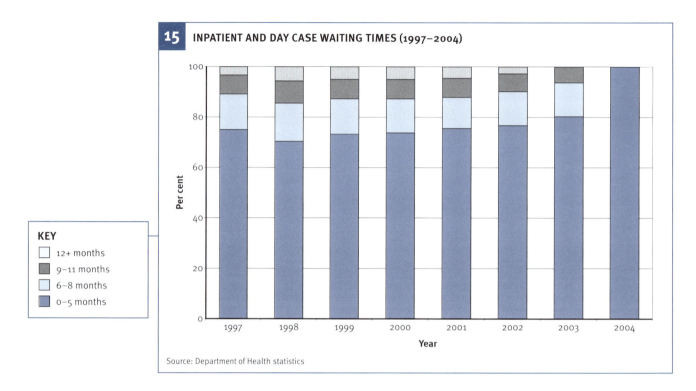

**15** INPATIENT AND DAY CASE WAITING TIMES (1997–2004)

**KEY**
☐ 12+ months
◼ 9–11 months
☐ 6–8 months
◼ 0–5 months

Per cent

Year

Source: Department of Health statistics

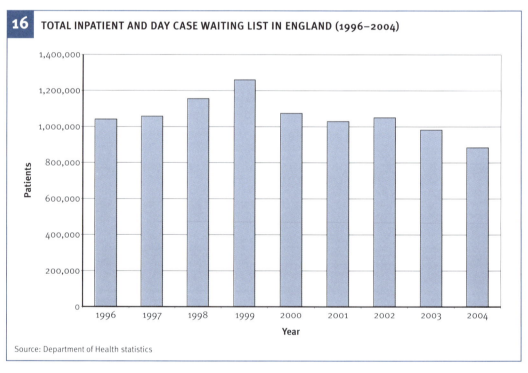

**16** TOTAL INPATIENT AND DAY CASE WAITING LIST IN ENGLAND (1996–2004)

Patients

Year

Source: Department of Health statistics

bypass grafts (CABGs) (*see* Figures 17 and 18 opposite), but waits for some procedures, for example implant of pacemakers, actually rose.

Attempts to increase day surgery rates appeared to have been modestly successful. The proportion of patients treated this way continued to rise, but the rate of growth began to level off towards the end of the period and was still some way short of the 75 per cent target (*see* Figure 19 on p 36).

**17**  **MEAN COMPLETED WAITS FOR SELECTED OPERATIONS IN ENGLAND (1998/99–2003/04)**

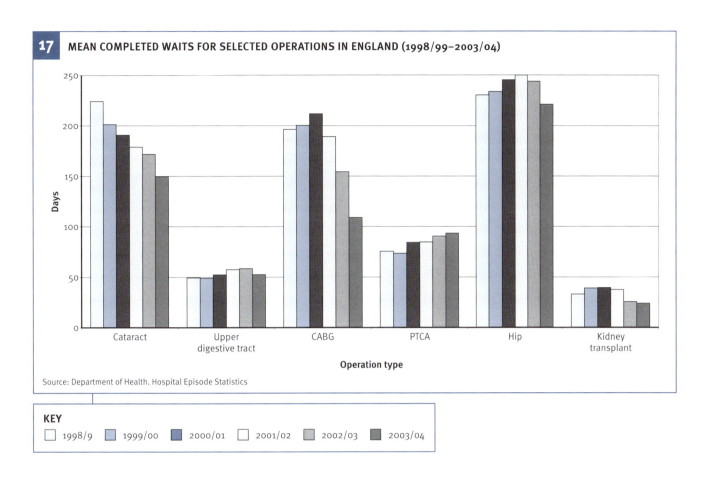

Source: Department of Health. Hospital Episode Statistics

KEY

☐ 1998/9  ■ 1999/00  ■ 2000/01  ☐ 2001/02  ■ 2002/03  ■ 2003/04

**18**  **MEDIAN COMPLETED WAITS FOR SELECTED OPERATIONS IN ENGLAND (1998/99–2003/04)**

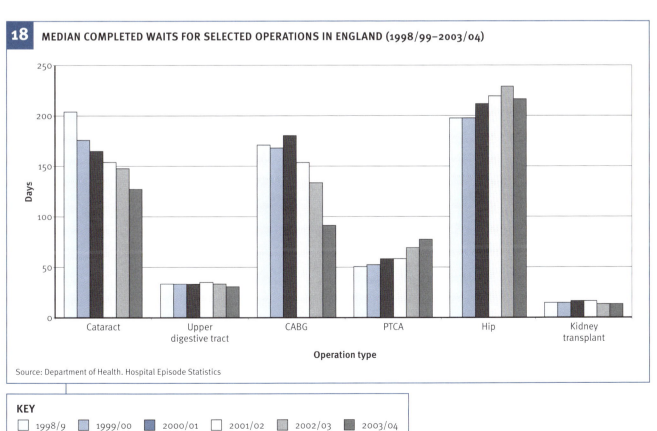

Source: Department of Health. Hospital Episode Statistics

KEY

☐ 1998/9  ■ 1999/00  ■ 2000/01  ☐ 2001/02  ■ 2002/03  ■ 2003/04

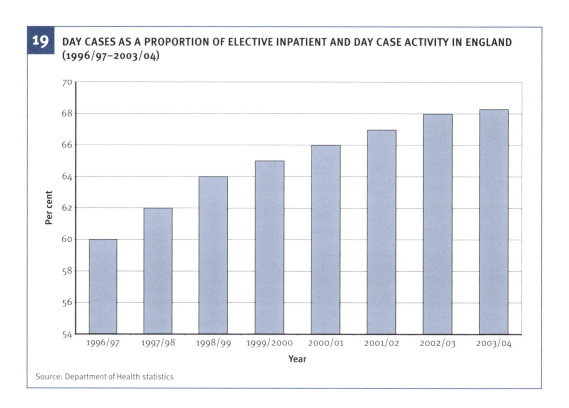

**19** DAY CASES AS A PROPORTION OF ELECTIVE INPATIENT AND DAY CASE ACTIVITY IN ENGLAND (1996/97–2003/04)

Source: Department of Health statistics

Other changes within hospitals suggested that their general operational efficiency was improving. The report *Winter and the NHS 2003–2004* (Department of Health 2004g) highlighted an increase in the number of hospital beds since 2000, improved discharge performance and better use of beds. One outcome had been a decline in the number of cancelled operations since the peak third quarter of 2000–01.

A report from the Audit Commission (2004) on health services in the community found that service redesign by PCTs to take advantage of GPs with a special interest had reduced waiting times, and possibly costs as well. Overall, it found that innovation had been limited.

The policies introduced during Phase 2 were primarily aimed at the NHS, although there was some evidence that the private sector was responding as well. The English private sector had been unsuccessful in its bids for the new treatment centres. As NHS waiting times came down, this sector perceived that its comparative advantage would decline. In response to this threat, some of the main private companies decided to become more effective competitors in what appeared to be a rapidly developing market for the provision of elective care to the NHS. In October 2003, for example, it was reported that for the first time the chief executive of General Health Group had offered to treat *all* long waiters for orthopaedic care (Timmins 2003a).

One result of the change in the market was a reduction in the price the NHS paid for operations. During the first policy phase and well into the second, the NHS was paying the private sector much higher prices than its own cost levels. By 2004 the government was able to announce that it was paying much less as the UK private sector reduced its own prices in response to the influx of foreign operators (Timmins 2004b).

However, the problem of long diagnostic waits remained, as far as it is possible to tell from the limited data available. A survey of trusts carried out by *The Sunday Times* in 2002 found evidence of some very long waits for magnetic resonance imaging (MRI) scans and other diagnostic procedures (*The Sunday Times* 2002). A survey carried out in north-west England in the same year (Pope and Sykes 2003) found that, while most waits were short, a small number of patients were waiting months for diagnostic tests.

In September 2004 the Royal College of Radiologists reported that the numbers waiting more than four weeks for diagnosis had doubled since 1998. At the same time, some cardiologists were claiming that this was also the case for heart patients as a direct result of the incentive payments doctors were being offered to refer promptly patients they suspected had heart disease (*Daily Mail* 2004). It seems that, as noted above, attainment of the initial access targets had been achieved at the expense of waiting at later stages in the care pathway (Robinson *et al* 2003).

Pressure on hospital resources was increased in other ways. Emergency admissions and A&E attendances grew steadily after 1997, continuing their upward trend (*see* Figure 20 below and Figure 21 overleaf).

The indirect effects of policies targeted on other objectives also made it hard to improve the elective care system. For example, measures to improve the overall quality of care absorbed surgical time especially at senior level, as did changes to the working hours of junior doctors in line with the European Working Time Directive and changes to their training regimes. More generally managers, including senior clinicians, were faced with a host of other policies, many of them complete with targets, which absorbed their energies and substantial chunks of their time. In particular, national initiatives such as *The NHS Cancer Plan* (Department of Health 2000j) and the *National Service Framework for Coronary Heart Disease* (Department of Health 2000k) made extensive claims on NHS resources. Hence, despite the political prominence of the waiting times targets and the emphasis on them in the performance management system, the overall policy context was not helpful.

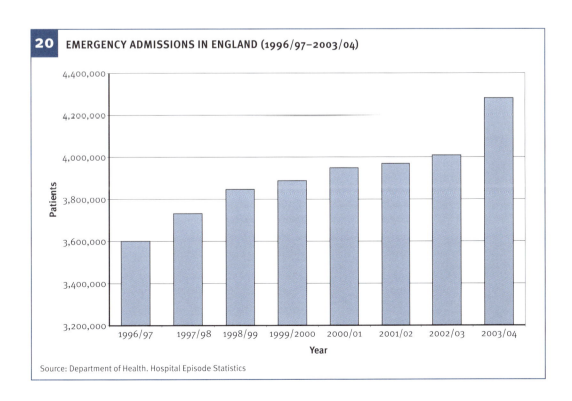

**20** **EMERGENCY ADMISSIONS IN ENGLAND (1996/97–2003/04)**

Source: Department of Health. Hospital Episode Statistics

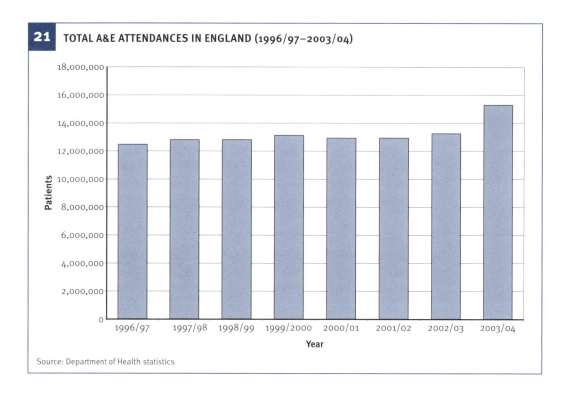

**21** TOTAL A&E ATTENDANCES IN ENGLAND (1996/97–2003/04)

Source: Department of Health statistics

## How were improvements in waiting lists and times achieved?

There is no way of demonstrating the links between particular policies and effects on the ground across the full range of the policies set out above. However, in the case of cataracts there does appear to be a clear link between the initiative taken in that specialty and the sharp reduction in waiting times achieved during this phase. The same is true for CABGs, which also benefited from a targeted initiative within the Choice programme. In the case of the national orthopaedic initiative, evidence of success did not emerge during this phase.

Overall, the total number of waiting list cases treated fell during this period (planned treatments continued to increase), which makes it hard to understand why the number waiting declined steadily during Phase 2.

A number of factors may have been at work. First, the number of some procedures, such as tonsillectomies, and dilation and curettages, which systematic reviews of the evidence had identified as being of low therapeutic value, may have declined. Such changes had occurred under the previous government as part of the development of evidence-based medicine.

Second, a number of procedures appear to have been reclassified as planned operations and others, primarily of a diagnostic nature, may have been reclassified and treated as purely diagnostic, in which case the waits would not be included in national figures. Others may have transferred to primary care settings.

Third, there was a marked reduction of about 100,000 a year in the numbers accepted for treatment (that is, put on the waiting list) between 2000–03 in comparison to the numbers accepted in the first policy phase. This drop in the flow of patients on to the list is sufficient in itself to explain why the numbers waiting fell consistently during this phase. However, it seems unlikely that the need for treatment declined during this period. This suggests that some degree of 'informal' demand management was in operation although precisely what is impossible to say on the basis of the available data.

Measures to improve capacity had little impact. Because it took time to establish the policies introduced from 2000 onwards, some of the main initiatives taken to implement *The NHS Plan* had not yet had a significant impact by the time *The NHS Improvement Plan* was published in 2004. In particular, the first wave of private sector contracts agreed following the bidding in 2002 had not started to have a major influence on the number of waiting list operations carried out. Use of the existing private sector did not expand to compensate for this (Timmins 2003b).

Many NHS treatment centres were operational by the end of 2004. However, their impact also fell short of expectations. Many found it hard to attract sufficient 'business' as patients, or GPs on their behalf, preferred to remain with their customary providers. By 2004 the treatment centres were running with spare capacity (Bate and Robert, forthcoming). In some cases, the resulting deficits threatened them with closure. A particular case in point was the Central Middlesex, which the government had often cited as a model for the modernised NHS.

The Choice programme was not fully underway by mid-2004. But within London there was evidence that the gains experienced in waiting times for heart surgery were a direct result of the pilot initiative, which had enabled those who would otherwise have waited longer than six months to be treated earlier. The trustees' report on the initiative declared the scheme to be a 'major success' (Department of Health 2003f, p 13). However, private sector and overseas providers made very modest contributions: about 1,000 patients a year have received treatment abroad and less than 60,000 within the UK private sector, of which 3,663 were treated in independent sector treatment centres (Department of Health official, personal communication 2005). Overall, the total was only a little higher than in 2000.

Finally, the impact of operational advice is hard to detect at national level. No independent audit of its overall effectiveness has been carried out, and as a result it is hard to assess the significance of the information that is available. The Birmingham evaluation report of the Cancer Collaborative identifies a number of improvements but also underlines the modest and possibly impermanent nature of the gains achieved (Robert *et al* 2003). In some cases, the impetus for improvement declined when the staff originally recruited to run the pilots left for other posts.

Throughout this phase *The NHS Plan* targets, the continual reinforcement of these targets by Department of Health officials and the star rating system left hospital trust boards in no doubt that a reduction in waiting times was the most important indicator against which their performance would be judged. Previous research for the King's Fund (Appleby *et al* 2004) has found that the minds of senior managers were focused, in some cases on an hour-by-hour basis, on what needed to be done to meet the current target. Sometimes this meant assessing which individual patients should be treated to ensure that the current target was not breached.

But while, in this sense, the targets worked, there were costs too. Under this pressure a number of hospitals were found to have 'fiddled the books' (National Audit Office 2001b; Audit Commission 2003b). The National Audit Office commented that (p 3):

> *Many of the investigation reports that followed allegations of inappropriate adjustments emphasise that a very strong message has been given, centrally and regionally, that delivery to achieve waiting line and waiting times targets are key priorities. While this does not in any way excuse inappropriate adjustment, the reports say that the adjustments were made in the context of pressure on trusts and particularly chief executives to meet key departmental targets.*

Some of these adjustments were relatively innocuous as far as patients were concerned: for example, in some cases managers suspended them from the list prior to the waiting list census being taken and then reinstated them. However, in other cases patients suffered: in some instances they were offered operations for times which they were unlikely to be able to accept, and if they refused the waiting clock was set to zero. Other cases of list adjustment could, to some degree, be attributed to poor information systems and, despite the salience of waiting times as a national policy issue, misunderstandings about how waiting times should be recorded (North Central London Strategic Health Authority 2004).

Another kind of 'cost' arose from the conflict between clinical and managerial targets. Clinicians consistently alleged that clinical priorities were distorted because, in their view, they had to place less needy patients ahead of more needy ones as a consequence of the approaching limits and deadlines. The National Audit Office (2001b) found that, out of 3,000 consultants surveyed, 20 per cent reported that distortion had occurred frequently and 32 per cent that it occurred occasionally. Similar findings were reported during the 1990s when the targets were much less demanding.

There is no way of knowing from this or similar surveys carried out in other countries just how important these conflicts were, and continue to be, in practice. There has been only a small amount of research on how clinical prioritisation works. What there is suggests that it remains very individualistic (for example, see National Audit Office 2001a).

There is therefore no 'gold standard' against which distortions can be measured. In the absence of this, the King's Fund has carried out an analysis of hospital episode statistics (Appleby et al forthcoming). This suggested that distortions due to the targets were small. There was also little evidence that unimportant procedures had been performed ahead of those that might be considered more important. It may therefore be that many of the consultants' complaints arose from their unhappiness about targets in general and interference with their clinical discretion.

This paper contends that the government was right to set targets for progressive reductions in waiting times since that sent a clear signal to the NHS as to what was desired of it. Some parts of the NHS needed this kind of signal: previous research published by the King's Fund (Appleby et al 2004) established that some consultants did not believe that long waits mattered to patients. Similarly, the studies of booked admissions by the University of Birmingham found a significant minority of consultants did not co-operate with their introduction. Without external pressure in some form, parts of the NHS would not have taken waiting seriously. Whether that indifference reflected the benefits of being able to offer some patients much more rapid treatment times in the private sector must remain a matter of speculation; this point is argued strongly by Light (2000).

## Overall assessment

The policies adopted by Labour during Phase 2 represent substantial progress over the previous period.

First, its overall policy objectives were significantly improved by the introduction of targets set in terms of a progressive reduction in maximum waiting times.

Second, the government brought a wider range of policies to bear on both the elective care system and the context in which it operated. In particular it acknowledged that capacity had to be increased if any improvement in waiting times was to be sustained and took active measures to ensure that it was. These measures took time to take effect, so in practice the main driver for improvement during Phase 2 remained the (improved) centrally imposed targets.

The range of technical advice available both to providers and to commissioners was vastly extended during Phase 2. But there were also clear limits to what had been achieved. The learning dissemination process appears to have been only partially successful. A report from the University of Birmingham on Phase 1 of the Cancer Collaborative (Robert *et al* 2003) showed that waiting times had been reduced from referral to start of definitive treatment for four out of the five cancers studied. The authors conclude (p 98):

> ... *some tumour types and some projects did demonstrate impressive progress for those patients who experienced the changes which were introduced. But as with other studies of collaborative and redesign methods, the variations on outcomes that occurred and the limited changes brought about in a number of projects, underline the continuing challenges of making the NHS more patient centred and tackling long standing capacity and cultural constraints.*

A report on the Orthopaedic Collaborative concluded that this collaborative had also brought about improvements but not on the scale envisaged at the outset (Bate *et al* 2002). It also identified 'gaps, flaws, omissions and weaknesses in the methods and processes used' that led the collaborative to undershoot the targets originally set.

Other research (Appleby *et al* 2004) found that some trusts did not have the necessary expertise to track or plan their own activity very far ahead. The University of Birmingham study also found a lack of relevant expertise. The final report on the booking programme (Ham *et al* 2002, p xv) concluded that:

> *This evaluation has shown that there are no magic bullet solutions to the challenge of booking. The main source of change and service improvement has to come from within each and every NHS organisation. Renewed effort now needs to be put into developing the staff and organisations that can embrace the kind of cultural change foreshadowed by* The NHS Plan. *No amount of guidance, support, hectoring or cajoling can substitute for the lack of capability and understanding among the staff delivering care to patients and the need to reshape the provision of services. It is this, together with the government's plans to increase capacity, that will unlock the potential demonstrated by the first wave pilots.*

This report also found marked differences between trusts. But perhaps the most disappointing finding, from the government's viewpoint, was that some of the pilots found it hard to sustain their initial progress and none of the pilot sites studied had managed to book all their day cases.

As this evidence shows, massive obstacles remained to introducing booking to all waiting list cases. In particular, the NHS still did not have the necessary expertise at the local level, despite the efforts of the NHS Modernisation Agency and its predecessors.

In a separate paper (McLeod *et al* 2003, p 1151) the authors of the Birmingham booked admissions studies conclude: 'Despite the progress made by the pilot sites, the NHS faces a substantial challenge in this area.' Their findings chime with other fieldwork carried out in late 2002 for the King's Fund (Appleby *et al* 2004). By that time most of the hospitals taking part in the research had not put in place the kind of integrated central management that a whole system view implied, although there were pockets of expertise. The extensive technical work from the NHS Modernisation Agency, the Audit Commission and the Department of Health, welcome though it was, did not appear to be effectively integrated either at national or local level.

Overall, the know-how and management systems required for effectively reducing waiting times were generally still not in place by mid-2004. These required both technical developments and the incentive to implement them. More importantly, they also required changes in working practices that are inevitably difficult to bring about. The national targets have helped to drive such changes in the past, and will continue to do so. But the evidence suggested that change on the ground would continue to be slow.

This raises the question as to whether the attempts made to change the way that the NHS provided elective care were radical enough. The Birmingham team summarised their experience of the collaboratives and the booked admissions programme as follows (Ham *et al* 2002, p 271):

> *The emerging conclusion from this and other UK studies (Bate et al 2001; Robert et al 2002) is that redesign methods and collaboratives have made a difference in the right circumstances. The extent of their impact and the sustainability of change is, however, crucially dependent on capacity, culture and leadership. In view of this, the more ambitious claims made for redesign should be interpreted with caution. Like previous fads and fashions in health care, there is a risk that redesign will be viewed as a panacea when all of the evidence suggests that it has a contribution to make as part of a more broadly based programme of performance improvement.*

Findings such as these and the need for more elective activity, identified in 2002, provided strong justification for the government's decision to seek out new providers and to create stronger incentives to change through the introduction of choice and PbR.

## Summary of Phase 2

By the end of Phase 2 the government had learned some key lessons:
- policies had to be sustained over the long term
- fundamental change in the existing system of providing elective care was necessary but hard to achieve
- new policies were required.

Could the government be confident by the end of Phase 2 that it knew what was required to meet the target it had set in 2000? By the time it issued new targets in 2004 success did seem within reach. But this section's analysis suggests that at least part of that success arose from changes within the elective care system – in particular the reduction in the flow of patients on to the waiting list – which were then, and remain now, poorly understood. They may have been affected by government policies but it is hard to establish the link.

Furthermore, the NHS treatment centre programme, although successful in terms of the number of units established, did not appear to be making the contribution expected of it. It is not clear why this was so, but one possible explanation might be that both patients and GPs have been generally content to stick with their local hospital even if waiting times are longer there (National Audit Office 2004; Bate and Robert forthcoming).

The evidence accumulated for Phase 2 also shows that improvements in access to initial consultations did not necessarily result in improvements across the patient journey as a whole. So although Phase 2 demonstrated a greater understanding of the nature of the problem to be tackled, it also revealed areas where it was poorly understood.

In brief:

- The objectives introduced during Phase 2 represent a vast improvement over those of Phase 1.

- The full mix of policies introduced during this phase had yet to take full effect by the middle of 2004, but by that date the numbers waiting overall and the number of long waiters had fallen sharply. There were signs that some policies, for example NHS treatment centres, were not working in line with expectations. However some specific initiatives, such as those directed at cataracts and heart disease, had achieved striking improvements.

- By the end of Phase 2 it was still not clear exactly how the elective care system as a whole was responding to the new range of policies. The inadequacies in the statistical coverage provided by official figures made it hard to distinguish between different explanations of the changes recorded in the numbers waiting and average waiting times.

# 4 Phase 3 (2005–2008 and beyond): the end of waiting?

This section covers the more recent policy initiatives introduced by the government to reduce, and potentially eliminate, waiting times. By mid-2004 the impact of the policies introduced in Phase 2 was limited. However, the section highlights that waiting lists were now falling rapidly. It sets out future challenges and analyses whether the government is likely to succeed in meeting its 2008 objectives.

*The NHS Improvement Plan* (Department of Health 2004a) set the NHS a new target for access to elective care. It stated that by 2008 no one should wait longer than 18 weeks from GP referral to hospital treatment. In setting a target in terms of the total time patients would have to wait, the government acknowledged that waiting for diagnostic tests and their results was just as important as waiting at other stages of the patient journey.

While the form of the new target represented an improvement over the old, it was viewed by commentators, and recognised by Department of Health officials, as challenging (*Health Service Journal* 2005). It required reductions in waiting times, as set by the existing targets, for initial consultation and treatment. It also required a reduction in the intervening diagnostic period where waits were sometimes very long, including waits between one consultant appointment and a subsequent one (although it is worth noting that neither of these waits is recorded in national statistics).

But if it could be achieved then, in the government's view, waiting for elective care would no longer be 'the main issue' (Department of Health 2004a, executive summary) and the NHS could move to other priorities, in particular 'provision of better support to people with illnesses or medical conditions that they would have for the rest of their lives'.

## New policies to finally eradicate unnecessary waiting?

Despite the demanding nature of the new target, there were several reasons for the government to feel confident.

First, the total number of people waiting for treatment continued to fall rapidly after publication of *The NHS Improvement Plan*. By the end of January 2005 the total was just over 861,000 (a fall of 100,000 over the year), the lowest figure for 16 years after five years of steady decline. Waiting lists had fallen in the past but never before over such a long period.

Second, the private capacity purchased in the first round of contracts was starting to come on stream, with more to come. *The NHS Improvement Plan* had suggested that up to 15 per cent of operations might be purchased from the private sector – much more than the first round of contracts would have produced. In the 2005 election manifesto the number was increased from the figure of 250,000 announced in 2003 to 460,000 operations a year and, while the government was careful not to make a specific commitment to a higher figure, the implication was that more would be purchased if required. At the same time, the emphasis changed from the purchase of needed additional capacity to the introduction of sufficient capacity to allow genuine competition.

In a speech at the NHS Confederation in June 2004 the NHS Chief Executive Sir Nigel Crisp stated, in spite of the evidence that NHS treatment centres were short of patients, that: 'We need more capacity so we can offer choice and there is some contestability. If everything is operating at 100 per cent that is stultifying' (cited in *Health Service Journal* 2004a, p 1). Later in the year the Secretary of State, John Reid, claimed the NHS purchasing of private capacity had 'smashed the consultants' "cartel"' (*Health Service Journal* 2004b). This had not been an explicit objective during Phase 2, but may well have provided some of the impetus to the decision made in 2002 to commission new capacity from overseas providers.

Third, contracts worth £3 billion over three years were agreed with the private sector in February 2005 (Department of Health 2005a) to overcome what had at last been recognised as a critical constraint on improving performance: a lack of diagnostic capacity. These contracts provide for massive increases in capacity – about one-third in the case of computerised tomography scans and 60 per cent in the case of endoscopies. This suggests that capacity should be available in the near future to overcome the diagnostic bottlenecks that would otherwise make it impossible to meet a target set in terms of all the waits patients experience on their journey through the system.

Fourth, the Choice programme was just beginning to take shape nationally, after successful pilots in London and elsewhere. *The NHS Improvement Plan* stated that by the end of 2005 all patients were to have a choice of five hospitals, including one private option. In early 2005, the Secretary of State announced that patients would have still more choice (Department of Health 2005b). Under these arrangements, as long as sufficient patients are prepared to travel to have their treatment, hospitals failing to make adequate progress towards the new waiting times target will see their waiting lists fall as (it is assumed) patients will choose shorter-wait hospitals. This will make it easier for poorly performing hospitals to reduce waiting times for their remaining patients and, because of the resulting loss of income, put pressure on them to improve their performance. Although the government decided in early 2005 to slow up the implementation of Payment by Results (PbR), it is still expecting it to be in place well before 2008.

Fifth, a major initiative was launched in 2004 aimed at reducing the emergency workload of hospitals (Department of Health 2004c). *The NHS Improvement Plan* had stated that, as waiting would soon cease to be the main issue for the NHS, the emphasis of health care policy would shift to long-term conditions. The department expected that this shift would reduce the numbers of people requiring emergency admission to hospital: all primary care trusts (PCTS) were set a new target of reducing emergency bed days by 5 per cent below the 2004 level by 2008. If this target is achieved then hospitals should find it easier to expand their elective activity. The contribution of other initiatives designed to reduce the workload of the acute hospital, such as the development of GPs and other professionals with special interests, should continue to grow.

Sixth, the number of foundation trusts is set to rise. In principle these should have greater capacity to respond to the opportunities to develop new or existing services that PbR should offer.

Finally, the National Orthopaedic Project, targeted on the most recalcitrant specialty, reported in early 2005 that a rapid reduction in the numbers waiting over six months had been achieved (Department of Health 2005c). Against this background the Department of Health was able to announce that the NHS as a whole was on track to meet the six month target by the end of 2005 (Department of Health 2005d).

If all the policies in place by the middle of 2005 work in line with government expectations, the NHS elective care system will shortly be transformed from the 'command economy' of the first two phases into a quasi-market economy. Hospital trusts will be put under unprecedented pressure from patients exercising choice (and taking the finance for their treatment elsewhere), other trusts offering quicker access and the private sector removing business out of the NHS altogether.

Against this background, the prospect is one of sustained progress towards the new target set in 2004.

## Will the new policies work?

There are several reasons why the new elective care system may not work quite as effectively as the government is clearly hoping. These are discussed below.

### Changes in the financial climate

The financial climate is becoming less favourable than it was in the years immediately after *The NHS Plan* (Department of Health 2000a) was published. Although spending on the NHS is still growing rapidly, trusts are experiencing strong cost pressures and purchasers are dealing with demand pressures (for example, from the introduction of new cancer drugs). By the end of the 2004–05 financial year a significant number of trusts were reporting deficits. A large share of the budgets of PCTs was being taken up by increases in the pay of NHS staff rather than by service expansion. The emergence of spare capacity within the NHS, in treatment centres and elsewhere, raised the possibility that the constraint on improving performance had switched from physical capacity to finance, at least in some parts of the country. In the medium term the prospect is that the NHS budget will cease to grow as rapidly as it has done since 2001. At the same time competing claims on this budget will continue to grow from services such as cancer and the other national service frameworks that are all guiding 10-year improvement programmes, which extend far beyond the current budgetary horizon.

There have also been signs that the pressure of emergencies, which had sabotaged efforts to improve waiting times in previous years, is re-emerging. While the reduced impact of winter pressures in recent years does owe something to better planning across health and social care services, it is also partly a result of the mildness and brevity of recent winters and the absence of a severe influenza epidemic. According to the *Chief Executive's Report to the NHS* in 2004 (Department of Health 2004d), total emergency admissions have risen by nearly 10 per cent since publication of *The NHS Plan*. Many of these are short stay admissions via accident and emergency (A&E) departments, but there is very little understanding of the reasons why this increase has occurred. There is therefore a risk that, despite the new policies, emergency admissions will continue to rise.

The government's hope is that new ways of managing chronic disease will reduce the pressures on hospitals by reducing the number of emergency admissions. There is strong prima facie evidence that admissions can be avoided by appropriate community interventions, but it is far from clear what the most effective means are of identifying those most at risk of admission and the interventions most likely to succeed in reducing that risk (Hutt *et al* 2004). It is likely to take some time before the full potential of such interventions is realised.

## Challenges to further reducing waiting times

The task facing the NHS is becoming progressively more difficult. Data presented in this paper have shown that it has proved far easier to make rapid reductions in *maximum* waits rather than average waits. This follows from the shape of the overall distribution of waiting times. As Figure 22 below shows, on average the distribution has an extended tail of long waiters – but not many fall into this category. As these long waits continue to be eliminated improvements will have to be made on the main part of the distribution where many more patients are involved.

Many are already waiting for short periods, that is less than two months, but reducing the waiting for the remainder demands a much greater effort than that expended to meet previous targets. The main effect of the progressive reduction of the maximum limits achieved by 2004 has been to squeeze up the distribution towards the left of Figure 22, that is, to redistribute waiting rather than reduce it overall. This fact goes a long way to explaining why maximum waits have fallen much more rapidly than average waits.

The 18-week target sets the NHS an additional challenge, far beyond what has already been achieved. To meet it requires complete elimination of all waits over a small number

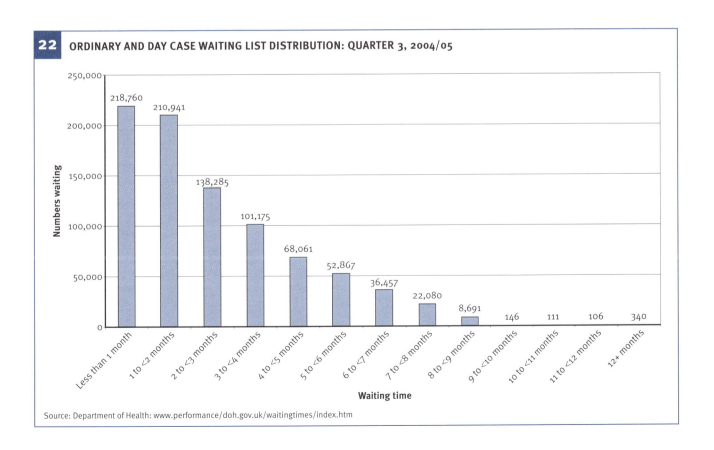

**22** ORDINARY AND DAY CASE WAITING LIST DISTRIBUTION: QUARTER 3, 2004/05

Source: Department of Health: www.performance/doh.gov.uk/waitingtimes/index.htm

of weeks at each stage of the process. There is very little information about the length of time people spend between first appointment and the decision to admit, but it is known that delays at this stage can be lengthy, particularly for non-urgent cases when diagnostic tests such as magnetic resonance imaging (MRI) scans are required. The measures announced should help to reduce these but they will not eliminate those delays that result from referral from one consultant to another. Although these form a significant and growing share of total referrals, there is no published data on the extra waiting time they give rise to – national data cover only the wait for the first appointment.

The elimination of these intermediary waits will require both the extra capacity that the government has commissioned from the private sector and effective management systems to ensure that the various stages of the patient journey are knitted together. Audit Commission findings (2003a) suggest that it cannot be taken for granted that the management and IT systems are in place to enable this to be done.

The NHS Modernisation Agency, through the collaborative programme and other measures, has actively promoted this kind of improvement in the past, but its role is being downgraded (Department of Health 2004h). Its work will continue at local level although, as the evidence cited in the previous section demonstrates, it has proved hard to introduce new systems of working rapidly across the NHS as a whole and also to sustain progress once it has been made.

## Inaccuracies in government estimates

The assumptions underlying the government's estimates of the extra capacity required may be proved wrong. These were initially set out in *Improvement, Expansion and Reform* (Department of Health 2002k): see National capacity assumptions 2002.

In the past, demand for hospital care has usually been forecast by simply extrapolating past trends. Very little analytic work has been carried out on the determinants of demand for elective care and some of the relevant factors, such as the rate of clinical innovation that expands the scope for treatment, are impossible to forecast with confidence. Moreover, any relationships that held in the past are unlikely to continue to hold in the very different elective care system that the government's policies are creating.

Two sources of uncertainty are likely to be particularly important. First, the more access times are reduced, the more activity will be required. The government has recognised that some people may switch from the private sector as waiting times reduce and has allowed for this in its estimates of how much extra capacity is required by assuming that many self-payers, about 200,000, will return to the NHS as waiting times fall. But the general scale of this effect remains uncertain. Research on the responsiveness of demand to shorter waiting times suggests that referrals from general practice will increase as waiting times are reduced (Harrison and New 2001; Goddard and Tavakoli 1998). Estimates of this effect vary from 0.1 to 0.3 per cent for every 1 per cent change in waiting time (Martin *et al* 2003).

By most standards this would be counted as an inelastic demand but, if waiting times were more than halved (as the current targets imply), the absolute effect would be substantial. However, as waiting times fall to levels not previously experienced in England it is doubtful whether these estimates, derived from a time when waiting was much longer, will continue to apply. Hence, the scale of this effect over the next few years must remain a matter for speculation rather than precise estimation.

---

**NATIONAL CAPACITY ASSUMPTIONS 2002**

- Differential between growth in elective activity and GP referrals of 3 per cent to ensure sufficient elective capacity to meet waiting time targets and offer choice.

- Day case rate increased to 75 per cent.

- Increased amount of activity taking place in primary and community settings to contribute to the national assumption of at least one million more outpatient appointments (around 10 per cent) take place in the community rather than in hospital.

- Sufficient bed capacity (including critical care) to ensure that bed occupancy drops to a level consistent with admitting emergency cases without delay.

- Support and incentives for routine delivery of fast and convenient access to primary care services for all patients by increasing and targeting resources in those practices or other service providers with particular resource, management or other developmental needs.

- Increase the amount of elective activity undertaken in dedicated facilities (including diagnostic and treatment centres) and non-NHS providers (including the private sector).

Source: Department of Health 2002k, Appendix B

---

It will depend, at least in part, on the second source of uncertainty: possible changes to treatment thresholds. Although the demand for elective care comes initially from individuals, in practice it is those they seek care from – their GP and subsequently the hospital consultant – who largely determine what care they receive. The wide variation in treatment rates between different parts of the country reflects the fact that clinical decisions embody a large subjective element. Falling lists combined with the new financial framework, which rewards higher levels of elective work, may well lead to a lowering of thresholds in the absence of any new initiative to define them more objectively.

In addition, thresholds may change for technical reasons. In recent years the most dramatic example of this has occurred within cataract surgery, which now may take place soon after a cataract begins to form, in contrast to the practice in earlier years of waiting until they were 'ripe'.

## Shortages of key staff

Although the government has succeeded in increasing the number of staff of all types working within the NHS (and hospitals in particular) there will probably remain shortfalls of key personnel (for example, in diagnostics and particularly radiology). A report from the Royal College of Radiologists (2002) argued that the number of radiologists should be doubled given the excessive workloads faced by some consultants. In February 2005 the Royal College of Surgeons published a paper warning that there was an incipient crisis in the supply of surgeons due in part to both the growing demands on consultants and a shortage of training posts. It has also been argued that establishing independent sector treatment centres would pose a threat to future training possibilities (Plumridge 2005).

Similarly, according to Cancer Bacup (2004), 45 per cent of cancer networks reported staff shortages as being the main obstacle to improving waiting times. The situation may worsen if, as predicted, the rate of retirement of senior staff increases over the next few years (Royal College of Surgeons 2005). The capacity planning guidance issued in May 2004 (Department of Health 2004i) acknowledged that shortages in a number of staff categories would be likely.

### Unanticipated responses to change

Both trusts and patients may not respond to recent policy changes in the way the government expects. The assumption implicit in the government's promotion of PbR and patient choice is that efficiency (and hence the output of the NHS's own elective care system) will rise as providers respond rationally to the incentives inherent in both policies.

What happens in practice will hinge on how trusts in different financial positions choose to respond in light of the new environment, and how the process of reallocation of workload takes places between them. PbR will be effective only if some trusts are enabled to expand and, crucially, wish to accept the risks of doing so. The scenario the government hopes to see realised is one where more efficient trusts steadily gain work and the overall cost of providing elective care falls. But they can respond in this way only by taking surgical and other specialised resources from other parts of the NHS, thereby reducing activity in the losing hospitals. It is therefore hard to predict what will happen to overall activity levels across the whole of the NHS.

In addition, PbR creates an incentive for hospitals to use their capacity to the maximum. While they might not positively seek to admit more patients as emergencies, they will have no incentive to reduce them.

As far as patients are concerned it remains uncertain how far the exercise of choice of provider will drive change. The London Patient Choice Project found that more than 50 per cent of patients were prepared to travel to another hospital (Dawson *et al*, 2004). But London offers a wide range of reasonably accessible hospitals. In other areas the scope for choice is much less: research outside London suggests that the majority of patients are not willing to travel to another hospital (Damiani *et al* 2004; Taylor *et al* 2004). The experience of NHS treatment centres also suggests a reluctance to move from local hospitals. Furthermore, a report from the National Audit Office (2004) found a general reluctance among GPs to exploit the potential for choice on behalf of their patients. The Department of Health's 2004 autumn performance report to Parliament (Secretary of State 2005) noted that between April and October 2004, of the 125,800 patients who had been waiting around six months and were offered the choice of faster treatment, only 19 per cent (24,300) took up the offer. International experience of choice schemes is in line with this experience (Brouwer *et al* 2003). Moreover, even where patients are prepared to travel the tendency for waits to even up will then reduce the incentive for others.

## Summary of Phase 3

Given the uncertainties described in this section, the outlook for continuing and sustained improvement in waiting times may be less favourable than recent improvements in performance might suggest.

This may seem an unduly pessimistic conclusion given the scale of the effort being devoted to improving waiting times. Evidence from other countries such as Germany and France suggests that waiting can be virtually eliminated if spending is high enough (Siciliani and Hurst 2003a). But even by 2008 England will be spending only as much on health care (as a proportion of GDP) as France did in 2001; France has been spending proportionately more than England since 1960.

Moreover, waiting times have emerged as a policy issue in recent years in countries such as Sweden and Canada, which spend as much as England will be spending in two to three years (Siciliani and Hurst 2003a, 2003b). In Scotland, which has enjoyed much higher levels of spending than England for many years, waiting times remain high relative to the new English target. Audit Scotland (2004) has reported an increase in both numbers waiting and average waiting times, as well as an apparent decline in total activity that could not be explained due to poor data systems. However, it is unlikely that the explanation is a lack of resources as a whole within the Scottish NHS. Waiting times in Wales and Northern Ireland have also been persistently longer than in England despite greater levels of funding over many years.

In brief:

- The objectives set during Phase 3 represented a further improvement over those from Phase 1: with the target set in terms of overall waiting time, patients' concerns about waiting were properly addressed and the scope for reductions in one part of the patient journey to be offset by increases in another was reduced.

- The range of policies in force during Phase 3 has reflected the initiatives taken in Phase 2 but with significant additions in respect of diagnostic and treatment capacity. They offer the prospect of further sustained improvements in performance and hence further falls in waiting lists and times. Nevertheless, significant challenges and risks remain:
  - other claims on the NHS budget continue to rise
  - to achieve the new target requires reductions in the majority of waiting times, not simply the longest
  - demand may rise faster than expected, in part due to the very success of the policies now being introduced
  - staff shortages remain
  - attempts to improve the efficiency of the elective care system may not be effective.

- Understanding of the nature of the elective care system improved with the abandonment of the backlog model. But the wide range of policies now coming into effect means that it is impossible to forecast how the elective care system will respond to them. The need for better monitoring is greater than ever.

While the government has made substantial progress in defining and tackling waiting lists and times, its objectives, policies and understanding of how the elective care system works do not yet amount to a fully worked out view of what is required. What more is needed is the subject of the next section of this paper.

# 5 What still needs to be done?

**This section asks whether the government will achieve its waiting time target of 18 weeks by 2008 and, if so, what still needs to be done. It analyses whether the right policies are in place, and suggests a better basis for future policy-making.**

As the government has progressed through the three policy phases described in sections 2 to 4, it has gradually developed its policy objectives and extended the range of policies designed to achieve them. The new targets reflect the public's concern about waiting times much better than those adopted originally. But, if the NHS does succeed in meeting the new target, will waiting become an endpoint after which policy should focus on ensuring that the target continues to be met? Or would it represent another staging post on the way to a yet more demanding policy? That requires a closer look at what the objectives of policy towards elective care should be and what form any new target should take. These are the subject of the first part of this section.

To achieve the new objectives the government has introduced a wide range of policies which, as they begin to take full effect, offer the prospect of substantial and sustained reductions in waiting times. But there are also grounds for thinking that the successes already apparent may be short-lived and that further progress may be more difficult to make than the government has allowed for. If there is a risk that the current policies will fail, what can be done to increase their chances of success? That requires a closer look at the policies that the government has adopted and what might be done to strengthen them, and also at the additional information and understanding that might assist in deciding what more needs to be done. This is addressed later in the section under the heading 'Are the right policies in place?' (*see* p 55).

## Moving in the right direction?

As it progressed from Phase 1 to Phase 3 the government improved how it expressed the reduction targets set for the NHS. The new formulation – combining waiting at all stages of the patient journey – reflects patients' actual experiences better than those that preceded it, and reduces the scope for measured waits to be improved at the expense of longer unmeasured waits for diagnosis.

Nevertheless, there remain a number of contentious issues that the government has yet to resolve if the objectives for access to elective care are to be properly framed.

### Should there be a national target?

This paper has argued that the government was right to set national targets as these have been essential for driving the necessary changes forward. For the same reason, they should be retained.

If national targets are retained, what form should they take? The government's new target correctly brings together all sources of waiting. But the form of the target – a maximum not to be exceeded by anyone – increases the risk of a clash of priorities between managers and clinicians. For example, what should happen in the case of a complex and difficult diagnosis that may take some time and a number of consultants to resolve? In addition, experience suggests that these kind of circumstances create intolerable pressures on managers, who must sometimes literally run around to ensure that a small number of patients are treated on time.

These difficulties can be avoided by slightly relaxing the target, as other countries employing similar policies have done. The King's Fund study (Appleby *et al*, forthcoming) of possible clinical distortions arising from attempts to meet maximum waiting times targets will suggest that, because the scale of the conflict is not great, a minor easing might have a significant effect in reducing the area of conflict.

## *Should the targets be more ambitious?*

The government introduced its modernised access programme drawing on work done in the United States. Put simply, this states that 'today's work should be done today'. Waiting should be minimal. The same argument has been put forward for elective care (Murray 2000).

In his first report on the future cost of the NHS, Sir Derek Wanless suggested an ambitious target of two-week waiting times at the inpatient and outpatient stages (Wanless 2002). But his report offered no reasoning in support of this; it also did not provide an estimate of the cost of achieving such a target.

Some research suggests that costs to the NHS may be reduced by more timely treatment (Saleh *et al* 1997). However, it could also be expected that the cost of reducing waiting would rise sharply as waiting fell towards zero because of the need to provide sufficient spare capacity to deal with unavoidable variations in demand. If there is scope for reducing the existing level of variation and adjusting the capacity available in line with the forecast changes, as some hospitals already do, then costs may not increase. Therefore, there would be no cost-based reason for not further reducing waiting times.

## *Is the target too ambitious?*

For patients referred with suspected cancer, minimising the length of time spent waiting to be seen and to be diagnosed is critical. But for others, such as those identified with early stage cataracts or whose symptoms are relatively minor, a few weeks of waiting time would be only modestly inconvenient, particularly if they are confident that the wait *will* be only a few weeks. Those patients who are diagnosed quickly and are informed that their condition is not severe or life threatening may also be prepared to wait. Research into the take-up of the London Patient Choice Project has shown that a significant number of people accepted a longer wait than they would have experienced if they were treated elsewhere than their local or first choice hospital – even though they were waiting for several months before being offered an alternative place of treatment (University of York, forthcoming). This suggests that the degree of discomfort they experienced was modest.

If the costs – in all senses of the term – to patients of waiting vary considerably and if, as in some cases, the costs are very low, then an 18-week overall wait for all conditions is arguably too ambitious. A better approach would be to match maximum waiting times to conditions, as already occurs with cancer and to a lesser degree with heart disease. This would also involve placing greater emphasis than current government policy has so far on getting clinical consensus on degrees of urgency between both patients and different clinical conditions.

A further option would be to allow patients to 'trade' longer waits for more convenient treatment days, times or locations. If patients wanted to be treated at a particular hospital then they might well choose to wait to be treated there, even if that hospital was popular. It would make no sense to penalise hospitals for allowing such voluntary waits to occur.

Alternatively, some patients could be given a choice between a certain but more distant date, and a less certain but nearer one. Those for whom waiting is not a concern might be content to wait for a longer time. The government has rejected this approach by emphasising the benefits to patients of having booked admission dates.

But there are costs attached to such a policy. If all admissions were booked that would effectively divorce the elective from the emergency side of the hospital, leaving the latter to deal with all the fluctuations in activity, including admissions and lengths of stay. A study of intensive care beds (Gallivan *et al* 2002) found considerable variability in length of stay after cardiac surgery: it concluded that these were incompatible with booking systems unless there was more spare capacity than currently existed (*see also* Jones 2001). The government has acknowledged the need for more capacity although there does not appear to be any published estimate of what it would cost to fully separate elective from emergency work.

There may be scope for reducing variations in demand, but where demand remains unpredictably variable then hospitals must either have spare capacity at some periods or find a way of creating slack on the elective side (NHS Modernisation Agency and NHS Confederation 2004; Rogers *et al* 2002).

### *Should targets be based on time alone?*

The focus on access times rests on an assumption, rarely made explicit, that the flow of referrals for elective treatment is itself unproblematic: that is, that the right people are being identified at the right time. If this condition does not hold then the pursuit of shorter maximum waiting times alone will not ensure that the fundamental NHS objective of equal access for equal need will be met (and this raises the question of *who* has benefitted from the reduction in maximum waits to date).

A National Audit Office (1997) study of cataract surgery in Scotland suggested that this was not the case for this particular procedure. Analysis of the utilisation rates of NHS services as a whole suggests that rates of surgery vary with social class, with lower social classes receiving lower rates of treatment (the relationship varies according to the type of surgery involved). Johnstone *et al* (1996) found that, for cardiology and cardiothoracic surgery, deprivation and the number of elective care episodes were inversely related. The opposite was true for ear, nose and throat (ENT), while for other specialities the relationship was less clear. There are also class-related variations in seeking access to care (National Audit Office 2004; Adams *et al* 2004). But, as this and other work demonstrates, the factors underlying variations in access are poorly understood, and hence successful policies are hard to devise (for example, *see* Majeed *et al* 2002).

Labour's first White Paper emphasised the equity objective across the NHS; it set in train a number of policies designed to promote both equality of access and quality of care. 'Fair access' formed one component of the national performance framework published in 1998, which was designed to enforce the principles set out in the White Paper (NHS Executive 1998b).

But, while these had implications for waiting lists, they did not represent a direct attack on them. That would require an explicit target for elective care in line with the objective of equal access for equal need: that is, equal treatment rates and treatment thresholds for similar populations.

In a speech discussing the results of the Department of Health's public consultation on its policies on patient choice (Reid 2003), the then Secretary of State directly addressed this point. Without discussing the reasons for variations in treatment rates in any depth – referring only to 'culture' – he argued that providing more and better information would create a level playing field. Subsequently he advocated that 'Choice is the route to equity as well as excellence' (Department of Health 2003g). Using this view, equity and choice are mutually reinforcing rather than conflicting goals.

*The NHS Improvement Plan* (Department of Health 2004a) acknowledges the need to provide financial support for travel costs if the benefits of choice of place of treatment are to be enjoyed by all the population. But, while potentially helpful, it is unlikely to be effective in reducing existing disparities and may even increase them if choice of hospital is widely taken up and hospitals, or some of their departments, close (Appleby *et al* 2003).

Support for physical access to hospital does not address the many other obstacles that influence whether or not patients seek treatment, or the degree of variation between GPs about whether or not to refer patients to hospital. Genuine equity of access will require a wide range of policies: patient choice will be only one.

Neither personal nor professional behaviour is easy to change but, given the commitment of the NHS to equal access for equal need, the next stage in the development of objectives for access to elective care must embody a commitment to progress in this direction.

## Are the right policies in place?

During its time in office the government has gradually extended the range of policies it has applied to the reduction of waiting times. By the start of the third policy phase it had begun to implement a process of radical reform based on the assumption that more capacity was required. It also reinforced its emphasis on improving the process through which care is delivered and reducing the cost of doing so through the introduction of competition.

The government has been right to adopt these policies as they offer the prospect of a sustained and substantial reduction in waiting times. But there are a number of risks to successfully implementing these policies, affecting both the demand for and provision of elective care. To improve the chances of success, the government needs to address these.

## Demand side risks

The main risk here is that demand will rise more rapidly than had been assumed when the 18-week target was set and insufficient capacity will be in place to deal with it. If this occurs as a result of medical advances that offer new forms of treatment, or better identification of need in the community, or because of switches from the private sector, then the right response would be to increase supply. The government has already allowed for that possibility by keeping its options open concerning the possible scale of contracts with the private sector.

But where demand results from shifts in treatment thresholds, extra capacity may not be the right response. Some form of demand management may be required instead.

The government has devoted little energy to the issue of clinical prioritisation and intervention thresholds. Despite the continuing complaints of the medical profession and the (limited) evidence that clinical priorities were being distorted, its policy was to fend off attacks rather than deal with the issue directly. Isolated examples apart, professionals made little contribution either. The Audit Commission (2003b) found, as have others (Appleby *et al* 2004), that the definitions of urgent and non-urgent remain highly variable. Similarly, the National Audit Office (2003) study of hip replacements found that there were considerable differences between surgeons as to whom they considered appropriate for treatment. Other work has identified ageism and other biases that are unacceptable on equity grounds (Levenson 2003).

The government may now be assuming that if the new targets are met the issue of conflicts in prioritisation will go away. But even within the new and more rigorous 18-week target there remains a need to distinguish between those who should be treated almost as emergencies and those who can safely wait for the whole of this period. Experience with the largely successful attempt to reduce cancer waiting times for initial consultation for urgent cases has shown that prioritisation remains far from perfect (National Audit Office 2004).

The need for defined access criteria has increased because of the introduction of Payment by Results (PbR), which provides a positive financial incentive for hospital trusts to increase activity levels. At present, at least as far as admissions from the waiting list are concerned, that is desirable up to a point. But, as waiting times fall, or as more capacity becomes available through policies directed at other types of admission, then the evidence suggests that thresholds will be modified to allow further admissions (Harrison and New 2001; Audit Commission 2003a).

Demand management may take many forms, ranging from comprehensive national schemes, such as that developed in New Zealand, to local systems based on the judgements of individual clinicians and lay people reinforced by budgetary controls over spending (Hadorn 1997a, b; Kipping 2002; Edwards *et al* 2003). Such measures may not be needed during the next four years, but they will be required in the medium to long term as activity increases to ensure that the (currently notional) elective care budget is effectively used.

## Supply side risks

During all three policy phases the supply of elective care within the NHS has proved problematic. The data presented in this paper have shown that, while the total number of elective operations has risen, the number of waiting list patients treated has not. The introduction of private sector capacity should reverse that trend, but there is a risk that NHS capacity will decline further. A number of measures can be taken to reduce that risk.

First, workforce issues require more attention. One of the main factors underpinning the government's decision to go outside the NHS for extra capacity was the inflexibility of the workforce due to the long training period required for surgeons and anaesthetists. The government has been slow to address this problem within the NHS itself. It was only as late as 2005 that proposals were put out for consultation on a new grade of surgical assistant almost precisely at the same time as the Royal College of Surgeons was identifying a potential shortfall in surgeon numbers. The same approach is required for other expensive skills in short supply. The government acknowledged the need for more flexibility in *The NHS Improvement Plan* (Department of Health 2004a). The proposals set out there for new training schemes for new roles must be vigorously pursued.

Second, the impact of PbR must be carefully monitored. PbR is far from being a settled system, so a firm forecast of its impact is not feasible. Its effect on activity levels, particularly those of 'failing' hospitals, must be carefully monitored and steps taken to ensure that activity overall does not decline if some hospitals do opt out of certain kinds of elective work.

Third, the potential for other sources of demand to continue to rise, particularly for hospital resources, must be addressed. The government has started to put in place policies designed to reduce emergency admissions but their impact on both hospital use and total costs remains uncertain (Hutt *et al* 2004). Work on how to identify those most at risk of admission is at an early stage (some of this is supported by the Department of Health). Much greater investment in this area is required.

Finally, the potential for improving the use of existing capacity should be examined further. Although the government was right to introduce new policies directed at a major expansion of treatment capacity outside the NHS itself, it cannot be confident that the balance between creating new capacity and using the existing capacity more efficiently is correct. If the NHS Modernisation Agency is correct in arguing that there remains vast scope for increasing efficiency within the NHS, then it is likely that the cost of increasing activity within the NHS will be lower than in the private sector. Without further analysis it remains unclear how effective the measures the Agency recommends will be in terms of cost reduction, and how the result would compare with buying further capacity from the private sector, if that proves necessary.

## A better basis for policy-making

The government's understanding of the elective care system has improved during the three policy phases. But important areas are poorly described in official statistics. The reasons why some of the changes that have been made since 1997 are also inadequately understood. The regular monitoring reports published by the Department of Health reveal very little about what is really going on.

Unlike the Treasury and its model of the economy, the Department of Health does not make available its own model of how the elective care system works. It is therefore not possible to judge directly how well founded the assumptions underlying the key decisions it has made are, for example on the amount of new capacity it has commissioned. But it is safe to say that the department has made only limited use of formally commissioned research.

Government papers from Phase 1 onwards have used the term 'whole systems' in recognition of the fact that 'everything connects with everything else', and official papers have set out some useful methodologies (NHS Modernisation Agency 2003; NHS Health Operational Intelligence Project 2002). But the ability to predict how the various elements of the elective care system interact with each other, or how the elective care system interacts with emergency care, remains limited.

This will never be easy to do, but progress is limited by lack of information or poor quality data. The whole system cannot be adequately described at national level: key elements such as the shift of activity to community settings or from 'counted' day procedures to 'uncounted' outpatient procedures are not known with precision. Only limited effort has been devoted to improving the statistical framework that would enable consistent measurement of the activity that is being carried out. For example, little is known of the numbers 'trapped' at the outpatient diagnostic stage of their journey through the system, vital information if the 18-week target is to be tackled.

This explains why it is not possible to set out what should be clear accounting relationships between referrals, decisions to admit, numbers treated, cancellations and deferrals. Although weaknesses of this kind are well known to Department of Health professionals and have been highlighted by the National Audit Office, no substantial effort has been made to address them. In addition, as the Audit Commission (2003b) has argued, the quality of the underlying data needs improving to ensure comparability between trusts and other providers.

The government might take the view that, with waiting lists falling and some waiting times reducing rapidly, there is no need for work of this kind – if the policy succeeds, that is enough. But to manage the downside risks set out above there is a continuing need for an effective monitoring system to identify more efficiently whether or not these risks are being recognised, and to define what measures are most likely to be successful in reducing them.

In summary, the following points are relevant when considering the government's objectives, policies and targets:

- The targets that the NHS is now trying to achieve by 2008 do represent a move in the right direction. But they do not represent an endpoint. Once achieved they need to be redefined to ensure that there is genuine equality of access for equal need and that they reflect the government's choice agenda.

- There are a number of measures the government can take to reduce the risks of the policies now in place not having the desired effect.

- There is a continuing need to improve the information available to monitor how the elective care system responds to these policies.

# 6 Recommendations

It is clear that the considerable efforts and resources devoted to reducing excessive waiting times in secondary care in the English NHS have, over the last five years, achieved a degree of success that at the outset many may have doubted. As this review has shown, such success was not the result of a policy 'magic bullet'. Large increases in funding, mainly targeted at waiting times reductions, have clearly been important, but by itself extra funding does not always produce results, as past experience has shown. Additional spending, coupled with a political commitment to reducing waiting times, a long-term target setting regime (and associated sanctions and rewards), and practical intervention to promote learning and disseminate proven methods for reducing waiting times, has managed to move the English NHS to a point where maximum waiting times for access to key parts of the secondary care system are now at a historic low.

Such success means that the English NHS has reached an important watershed on waiting times, not least with regard to the sustainability of the achievements so far and the impact on waiting times of new policies such as patient choice and Payment by Results (PbR).

Three broad issues need to be addressed:
- the objectives of waiting list policy
- the policies to achieve these objectives
- the development of an understanding of the system that gives rise to waiting.

## Objectives

The objectives adopted in 2004 will continue to drive the NHS in the right direction. But they need to be developed further:

- As the new 18-week headline target is approached, more emphasis should be given to reducing differences in access levels between similar populations. This will require detailed examination of the scale of current variations, the reasons for their existence and the policies most likely to be effective in reducing them.

- Vastly reduced waiting times highlights a deeper issue concerning clinical priorities and treatment thresholds. Much more work is needed in these areas as part of a more systematic programme of demand management designed both to reduce the risk of demand responding inappropriately to shorter waiting times and to ensure the efficient use of NHS resources.

- The costs – and benefits – of reducing waits beyond the current targets should be estimated in terms of the health (and perhaps other) benefits to patients, and the costs and benefits to the NHS, with a view to establishing whether or not it is worth setting even more demanding objectives for Phase 4 of policy.

As patient choice develops, and if patients, through their choices, become more active in contributing to improvements in health services, central target/objective setting becomes less relevant and a more complicated set of 'objectives' (in effect the outcomes of patients' choices) may emerge as a result of trade-offs patients make between, for example, high quality providers and short wait providers. The objectives for access to elective care will have to shift from centrally imposed universal targets to targets that reflect the preferences of individuals.

## Policies

The present mix of policies, given adequate resources, has the capacity to deliver the reductions in waiting the government is currently aiming for, but its policies are nevertheless subject to a number of demand and supply side risks. To reduce the downside risks the government should:

- carefully monitor the impact of PbR and adjust the payment system if it becomes apparent that it is leading to a net reduction in the number of NHS operations or to an increase in emergency admissions
- pursue the agenda already set out for improving the supply of scarce skills (for example, in anaesthesia and radiology)
- invest more in the research and monitoring required to ensure that the policies it is introducing for the better management of long-term conditions are effective in reducing hospital admissions and in reducing overall NHS costs
- take steps to ensure the right balance between new capacity and better use of existing capacity, and between further ring-fencing of elective care and better management of elective and emergency flows within individual hospitals.

## Understanding the system

There are a number of weaknesses in the existing monitoring framework and a lack of understanding of the effect of new policies on the elective care system. In light of this, the government should consider the following:

- There needs to be improved monitoring and management systems nationally and locally, and better costing and financial control of patient journeys and demand. The model implicit in current policies should be made explicit and, like the Treasury model of the economy, open for everyone to assess and use to make their own forecasts.

- There should be greater consistency between the various sources of data describing the elective care system so that a reliable picture can be presented of the stocks and flows in the system.

# Annexe 1 The elective care system

In the English NHS most patients gain access to elective care within the NHS by moving along the pathway set out in Figure 3.

**3** **A PATIENT'S JOURNEY (OR THE 'PATIENT PATHWAY') THROUGH THE HEALTH SYSTEM**

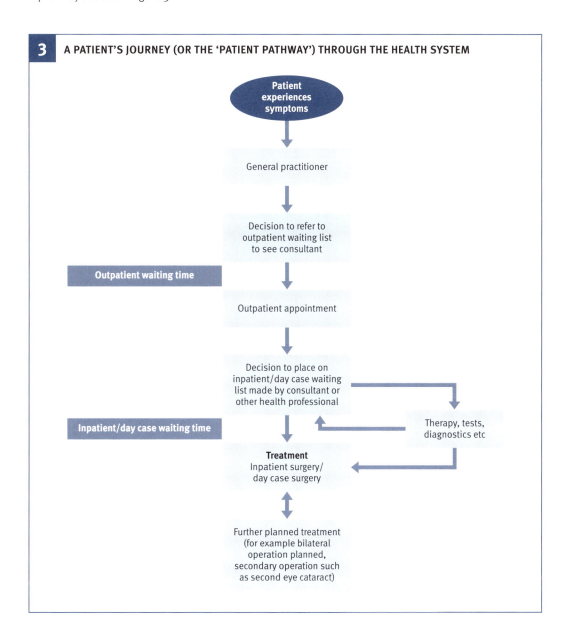

The patient takes the first step along the pathway when deciding to consult a GP (in some other countries patients can skip this first step and go directly to a hospital consultant or equivalent). Subsequently both GPs and hospital consultants act as gatekeepers: if both 'open' the gate, the patient is duly treated some time after the initial consultation.

Changes introduced by the government and developments in individual trusts have modified the pathway in a number of ways: for example, some professionals, such as optometrists, may refer directly to a hospital consultant and bypass the GP. Within hospitals, alternative routes to the pathway have been created, such as clinics run by nurses within orthopaedic departments. Potentially more important than all of these, introduction of patient choice will mean that patients and their GPs will be faced with a range of pathways leading to different hospitals.

While the pathway diagram provides a useful snapshot of the elective care systems, it does not provide any information as to how it works, that is, what factors determine the decisions that are made at each of the main stages by which access to care is achieved.

The key point is that these decisions embody a wide degree of discretion and individual judgement even where, as with cancer, national guidelines exist.

Among the factors that may influence them is the knowledge each decision-maker has of the situation in other parts of the elective care system and of the wider environment, including financial and other pressures. GPs may modify their decisions in light of what they know about waiting times for consultation, and consultants may modify their decisions in light of what they know about the length of their own waiting list and the pressures being brought to bear to reduce it and improve waiting times. Patients themselves determine when to enter the system and whether to remain within the NHS if they consider waiting times unacceptable.

One important implication of the discretion that exists is that waiting lists and times may vary because of the way that principal actors – patients, GPs and hospital consultants – respond to the information they have about the state of the elective care system around them. This may mean that GPs reduce their referral rate when waiting times are long and manage their patients within their own practice or send them to other treatment options. Similarly, it may mean that consultants under pressure to meet targets slow down the rate at which they accept patients for treatment, either by modifying their treatment thresholds or by deferring a decision to treat until after a further consultation.

These areas of professional discretion mean that waiting lists may fall or rise even when there is no change in the number of patients seeking treatment and in the number of operations being carried out. Only a modest amount of research has been conducted into the importance of these effects; however there is a particular lack of work on the response of hospital consultants to the incentives and pressures they face.

In the new elective care system the government is establishing, patients and GPs will enjoy more discretion as to how care is accessed. Consultants will have less discretion, since their control over the flow of patients coming to them will be reduced. At the same time, they and the hospitals within which they work will have to deal with a new set of choices: should they try to expand activity if their capacity is full or should they contract if they have spare capacity?

# Bibliography

Adams J, White M, Forman D (2004). 'Are there socioeconomic gradients in stage and grade of breast cancer at diagnosis? Cross-sectional analysis of UK cancer registry data'. *British Medical Journal*, vol 329, pp 142–43.

Appleby J, Boyle S, Devlin N, Harley M, Harrison A, Thorlby R (forthcoming). 'Do English NHS waiting times targets distort treatment priorities in orthopaedics?'. *Journal of Health Services Research and Policy*.

Appleby J, Boyle S, Devlin N, Harley M, Harrison A, Locock L, Thorlby R (2004). *Sustaining Reductions in Waiting Times: Identifying successful strategies, final report to the Department of Health*. London: King's Fund.

Appleby J, Dixon J (2004). 'Patient choice in the NHS'. *British Medical Journal*, vol 329, pp 61–62.

Appleby J, Harrison A, Dewar S (2003). 'Patient choice in the NHS'. *British Medical Journal*, vol 326, pp 407–8.

Audit Commission (2004). *Quicker Treatment Closer to Home: Primary care trusts' success in redesigning care pathways*. London: Audit Commission.

Audit Commission (2003a). *Achieving The NHS Plan: Assessment of current performance, likely future progress and capacity to improve*. London: Audit Commission.

Audit Commission (2003b). *Waiting List Accuracy*. London: Audit Commission.

Audit Commission (2003c). *Waiting for Elective Admission*. London: Audit Commission.

Audit Commission (2002). *Access to Care: Ear, nose and throat and audiology services*. London: Audit Commission.

Audit Commission (2001). *Day Surgery: Review of national findings*. London: Audit Commission.

Audit Commission (1998). *Day Surgery Follow Up: Progress against indicators from 'A Short Cut to Better Services'*. London: Audit Commission.

Audit Commission (1990). *A Short Cut to Better Services: Day surgery in England and Wales*. London: Her Majesty's Stationery Office.

Audit Scotland (2004). *An Overview of the Performance of the NHS in Scotland*. Edinburgh: Audit Scotland.

Bate P, Robert G (forthcoming). *Build It and They Will Come – Or Will They? Choice, policy paradoxes and the case of NHS treatment centres*.

Bate P, Robert G, McLeod H (2002). *Report on the 'Breakthrough' Collaborative Approach to Quality and Service Improvement Within Four Regions of the NHS*. Birmingham: Health Services Management Centre, University of Birmingham.

BBC News (2005). 'NHS targets to change'. 30 March. htttp://news.bbc.uk/go/pr/fr/-/hi/uk_politics/4393291.stm

Bensley D, Halsall J, McIlwain C, Scott L (1997). *Total Booking Systems for Elective Admissions*. Internal Department of Health report.

British Medical Association (1998). *Waiting List Prioritisation Scoring Systems: A discussion paper*. London: British Medical Association.

Brouwer W, van Exel J, Hermans B, Stoop A (2003). 'Should I stay or should I go? Waiting lists and cross border care in the Netherlands'. *Health Policy*, vol 63, pp 289–98.

Burrows N, Norris P (2004). 'More than skin deep'. *Health Service Journal*, 21 October, pp 24–25.

Cancer Bacup (2004). *Living With Cancer: Waiting for treatment*. London: Cancer Bacup.

Cant PJ, Yu DSL (2000). 'Impact of the "2 week wait" directive for suspected cancer on service provision'. *British Journal of Surgery*, vol 87, 8, pp 1082–86.

Clinical Standards Advisory Group (1993). *District Elective Surgery: Access to and availability of services*. London: Her Majesty's Stationery Office.

Cocker S, Elliott L (2003). 'The skin trade'. *Health Service Journal*, 13 February, p 32.

Daily Mail (2004). 'Heart patients dying as waiting lists for a scan grow, say doctors'. *Daily Mail*, September 27.

Damiani M, Proper C, Dixon J (2005). 'Mapping choice in the NHS: cross-sectional study of routinely collected data'. *British Medical Journal*, vol 330, pp 284–87.

Dawson D, Jacobs R, Martin S, Smith P (2004). *Evaluation of the London Patient Choice Project: System wide impacts. Final report*. York: Centre for Health Economics.

Department of Health (2005a). *Quicker scans: endoscopies and imaging for NHS patients*. Press Release 2005/0064. London: Department of Health.

Department of Health (2005b). *Choice of hospital for planned operations expanded – Reid*. Press Release 2005/0122. London: Department of Health.

Department of Health (2005c). *The National Orthopaedic Project: Faster access for NHS patients*. London: Department of Health.

Department of Health (2005d). *NHS on track to meet December 2005 target that no patient will wait more than six months for surgery*. Press Release 2005/0164. London: Department of Health.

Department of Health (2005e). *20,000 treated since start of pioneering treatment centre programme*. Press Release 2005/0005. London: Department of Health.

Department of Health (2004a). *The NHS Improvement Plan: Putting people at the heart of public services*. London: The Stationery Office.

Department of Health (2004b). *10 high impact changes that could transform NHS patient services*. Press Release 2004/0327. London: Department of Health.

Department of Health (2004c). *New reward scheme will mean faster treatment for patients*. Press Release 2004/0258. London: Department of Health.

Department of Health (2004d). *Chief Executive's Report to the NHS: May and October 2004*. London: Department of Health.

Department of Health (2004e). *The NHS Cancer Plan and the New NHS: Providing a patient-centred service*. London: Department of Health.

Department of Health (2004f). *Winning the War on Heart Disease: The National Service Framework for Coronary Heart Disease – progress report*. London: Department of Health.

Department of Health (2004g). *Winter and the NHS 2003–2004*. London: Department of Health.

Department of Health (2004h). *The Future Direction of the NHS Modernisation Agency*. London: Department of Health.

Department of Health (2004i). *Access Capacity Planning Guidance for the Period 2006/07–2007/08*. London: Department of Health.

Department of Health (2003a). *250,000 NHS patients to receive quicker treatment in new treatment centres*. Press Release 2003/0337. London: Department of Health.

Department of Health (2003b). *New £56 million drive to reduce blindness and impaired vision*. Press Release 2003/0206. London: Department of Health.

Department of Health (2003c). *Milburn sets out expansion plans for NHS Choice: success of heart surgery pilots means patient choice goes nationwide*. Press Release 2003/0053. London: Department of Health.

Department of Health (2003d). *Choice of Hospital: Guidance for Primary Care Trusts, NHS Trusts and Strategic Health Authorities*. London: Department of Health.

Department of Health (2003e). *New roles for nurses and GPs to expand primary care and drive down waiting lists*. Press Release 2003/0174. London: Department of Health.

Department of Health (2003f). *Heart Choice Initiative: Trustees' report July 2002/July 2003*. London: Department of Health.

Department of Health (2003g). *A flexible, fair NHS for all patients all the time*. Press Release 2003/0504. London: Department of Health.

Department of Health (2002a). *Delivering The NHS Plan: Next steps on investment, next steps on reform*. London: The Stationery Office.

Department of Health (2002b). *A new role for overseas and independent healthcare providers in England*. Press Release 2002/0283. London: Department of Health.

Department of Health (2002c). *Using Overseas Clinical Teams to Reduce Waiting Times: Guidance for NHS trusts*. London: Department of Health.

Department of Health (2002d). *Growing Capacity: A new role for external healthcare providers in England*. London: Department of Health.

Department of Health (2002e). *Thousands of patients to benefit from day surgery expansion*. Press Release 2002/0354. London: Department of Health.

Department of Health (2002f). *Day Surgery: Operational guide*. London: Department of Health.

Department of Health (2002g). *Improving Orthopaedic Services*. London: Department of Health.

Department of Health (2002h). *Extra capacity to be used to speed up heart surgery for NHS patients.* Press Release 20002/0118. London: Department of Health.

Department of Health (2002i). *Choice extended to benefit thousands more NHS patients: heart surgery leads way in delivering NHS choice.* Press Release 2002/04040. London: Department of Health.

Department of Health (2002j). *£66 million intermediate care help to speed up transfers from hospital.* Press Release 2000/01117. London: Department of Health.

Department of Health (2002k). *Improvement, Expansion and Reform: The next three years – priorities and planning framework 2003–2006.* London: Department of Health.

Department of Health (2001a). *Extending Choice for Patients: A discussion document: proposals for pilot schemes to improve choice and provide faster treatment.* London: Department of Health.

Department of Health (2001b). *National Booked Admissions Programme: Moving to mainstream.* Health Service Circular 2001/009. London: Department of Health.

Department of Health (2001). *2001/2002 arrangements for whole system capacity planning.* Health Service Circular 2001/014. London: Department of Health.

Department of Health (2000a). *The NHS Plan: A plan for investment, a plan for reform.* London: The Stationery Office.

Department of Health (2000b). *Tackling Outpatient Waiting Times: A new approach.* London: Department of Health.

Department of Health (2000c). *Booked admissions work in the NHS.* Press Release 2000/0669. London: Department of Health.

Department of Health (2000d). *For the Benefit of Patients: A concordat with the private and voluntary health care provider sector.* London: Department of Health.

Department of Health (2000e). *Denham announces details of faster cataract services.* Press Release 2000/0077. London: Department of Health.

Department of Health (2000f). *Local schemes for better cataract services published.* Press Release 2000/0388. London: Department of Health.

Department of Health (2000g) *All hospital trusts to offer booked appointments.* Press Release 2000/0533. London: Department of Health.

Department of Health (2000h). *Winter 2000/01: Capacity planning for health and social care.* London: Department of Health.

Department of Health (2000i). *Shaping the Future NHS: Long term planning for hospitals and related services (National Beds Inquiry).* London: Department of Health.

Department of Health (2000j). *The NHS Cancer Plan: A plan for investment, a plan for reform.* London: Department of Health.

Department of Health (2000k). *National Service Framework for Coronary Heart Disease.* London: Department of Health.

Department of Health (2000l). *NHS delivers on breast cancer target.* Press Release 2000/0148. London: Department of Health.

Department of Health (1999a). *20 million pound boost to reduce waiting lists and waiting times*. Press Release 1999/0097. London: Department of Health.

Department of Health (1999b). *John Denham announces £30 million to step up war on NHS waiting*. Press Release 1999/0512. London: Department of Health.

Department of Health (1999c). *Airline-style booking system for NHS to expand*. Press Release 1999/0230. London: Department of Health.

Department of Health (1998a). *Rewards for hitting waiting list targets*. Press Release 1998/0139. London: Department of Health.

Department of Health (1998b). *Modernising Health and Social Services: National priorities guidance 1999/00–2001/02*. London: Department of Health.

Department of Health (1998c). *Breast cancer waiting times: Achieving the target*. Health Service Circular 1998/242. London: Department of Health.

Department of Health (1998d). *Waiting lists fall by 45,000 – supertanker turns*. Press Release 1998/0349. London: Department of Health.

Department of Health (1997). *The New NHS*. London: The Stationery Office.

Department of Health (1996). *A Service with Ambitions*. London: The Stationery Office.

Department of Health and Social Security (1981). *Orthopaedic Services: Waiting time for outpatient appointments and inpatient treatment*. London: Her Majesty's Stationery Office.

Derrett S, Devlin N, Hansen P, Herbison P (2003). 'Prioritising patients for elective surgery: a prospective study of clinical priority assessment criteria in New Zealand'. *International Journal of Technology Assessment in Health Care*, vol 19, 1, pp 91–105.

Derrett S, Devlin N, Harrison A (2002a). 'Waiting in the NHS: Part 1 – diagnosis'. *Journal of the Royal Society of Medicine*, vol 95, 5, pp 223–26.

Derrett S, Devlin N, Harrison A (2002b). 'Waiting in the NHS: Part 2 – a change of prescription'. *Journal of the Royal Society of Medicine*, vol 95, 6, pp 280–83.

Derrett S, Paul C, Morris JM (1999). 'Waiting for elective surgery: effects of health-related quality of life'. *International Journal for Quality in Health Care*, vol 11, 1, pp 47–57.

Dunn E, Black C, Alonso J, Norregaard JC, Anderson GF (1997). 'Patients' acceptance of waiting for cataract surgery: what makes a wait too long?'. *Social Science and Medicine*, vol 44, 11, pp 1603–10.

Edwards RT, Boland A, Wilkinson C, Cohen D, Williams J (2003). 'Clinical and lay preferences for the explicit prioritisation of elective waiting lists: survey evidence from Wales'. *Health Policy*, vol 63, pp 229–37.

Galasko C (2000). 'Seven reasons why surgical consultants have their hands tied when it comes to increasing productivity'. *Health Service Journal*, 8 August, pp 23–24.

Gallivan S, Utley M, Treasure T, Valencia O (2002). 'Booked admissions and hospital capacity: mathematical modelling study'. *British Medical Journal*, vol 324, pp 280–82.

Gallivan S, Utley M (2001). 'Counting the cost of not allowing for spare capacity in the NHS'. *Health Service Journal*, 15 November, pp 20–21.

Goddard JA, Tavakoli M (1998). 'Referral rates and waiting lists: some empirical evidence'. *Health Economics*, vol 7, pp 545–49.

Hadorn DC, Holmes AC (1997a). 'The New Zealand priority criteria project: Part 1 – overview'. *British Medical Journal*, vol 314, pp 131–34.

Hadorn DC, Holmes AC (1997b). 'The New Zealand priority criteria project: Part 2 – coronary artery bypass graft surgery'. *British Medical Journal*, vol 314, p 135–38.

Ham C, Kipping R, McLeod H, Meredith P (2002). *Capacity, Culture and Leadership: Lessons from experience of improving access to hospital services*. Birmingham: Health Services Management Centre, University of Birmingham.

Hamblin R, Harrison A, Boyle S (1998a). 'How long was it for you?'. *Health Management*, June, pp 12–13.

Hamblin R, Harrison A, Boyle S (1998b). *Accessing Elective Care*. Unpublished paper available from the authors.

Hamblin R, Harrison A, Boyle S (1997). 'The supertanker's not for turning'. *The Lancet*, vol 350, pp 1493–94.

Hamilton BH, Hamilton VH, Mayo NE (1996). 'What are the costs of queuing for hip fracture surgery in Canada?'. *Journal of Health Economics*, vol 15, pp 161–85.

Harley M (2001). 'Bone of Contention'. *Health Service Journal*, 17 May.

Harrison A, New B (2001). *Access to Elective Care: What should really be done about waiting lists*. London: Kings Fund.

Harry LE, Nolan JF, Elender F, Lewis F (2000). 'Who gets priority? Waiting list assessment using a scoring system'. *Annals of the Royal College of Surgery of England*, vol 82, pp 186–88.

*Health Service Journal* (2005). 'Waiting target in early trouble'. *Health Service Journal*, 21 June, p 6.

*Health Service Journal* (2004a). 'Spare capacity vital to a system built round choice'. June. Accessed at www.hsj.co.uk

*Health Service Journal* (2004b). 'Bullish Reid claims victory over "cartels"'. *Health Service Journal*, 7 October, p 5.

Hemingway H, Crook AM, Feder G, Dawson JR, Timmis A (2000). 'Waiting for coronary angiography: is there a clinically ordered queue?'. *The Lancet*, vol 355, pp 985–86.

Hill L, Rutter I (2001). 'Cut to the quick'. *Health Service Journal*, 4 October.

House of Commons Health Committee (1991). *Public Expenditure on Health Services: Waiting lists*. London: Her Majesty's Stationery Office.

House of Commons Public Accounts Committee (2002a). *Inpatient and Outpatient Waiting in the NHS*. London: The Stationery Office.

House of Commons Public Accounts Committee (2002b). *Inappropriate Adjustments to NHS Waiting Lists*. London: The Stationery Office.

House of Commons Welsh Affairs Committee (1991). *Elective Surgery*. London: Her Majesty's Stationery Office.

Hutt R, Rosen R, McCauley J (2004). *Case-managing Long-term Conditions: What impact does it have on the treatment of older people?*. London: King's Fund.

Johnstone F, Lucy J, Scott-Samuel A, Whitehead M (1996). *Deprivation and Health in North Cheshire: An equity audit of health services*. Liverpool: Liverpool Public Health Observatory.

Jones R (2001). 'Quick quick slow'. *Health Service Journal*, 25 October, pp 20–23.

Jonsdottir H, Baldursdottir L (1998). 'The experience of people awaiting coronary artery bypass graft surgery: the Icelandic experience'. *Journal of Advanced Nursing*, vol 27, pp 68–74.

King's Fund (2005). *An Independent Audit of the NHS under Labour (1997–2005)*. London: King's Fund.

Kipping R, Meredith P, McLeod H, Ham C (2000). *Booking Patients for Hospital Care: A progress report*. Birmingham: Health Services Management Centre, University of Birmingham.

Kipping R, Robert G, McLeod H, Clark J (2002). *A Review of Priority Scoring and Slot Systems for Elective Surgery*. Birmingham: Health Services Management Centre, University of Birmingham.

Labour Party (2005). *Waiting Times: Forward not back*. London: Labour Party.

Levenson R (2003). *Auditing Age Discrimination: A practical approach to promoting age equality in health and social care*. London: King's Fund.

Lewis R, Collins R, Flynn A, Emmans Dean M, Nyers L, Wilson P, Eastwood A (2005). 'A systematic review of cancer waiting time audits'. *Quality and Safety in Health Care*, vol 14, pp 62–66.

Light D (2000). 'The two tier syndrome behind waiting lists'. *British Medical Journal*, vol 320, pp 1349–50.

Majeed A, Eliahoo J, Bardsley M, Morgan D, Bindman AB (2002). 'Variation in coronary artery bypass grafting, angioplasty, cataract surgery and hip replacement rates among primary care groups in London: association with population and practice'. *Journal of Public Health Medicine*, vol 24, 1, pp 21–26.

Martin S, Jacobs R, Rice N, Smith P (2003). *Waiting Times for Elective Surgery: A hospital based approach – project report*. York: Centre for Health Economics.

McLeod H, Ham C, Kipping R (2003). 'Booking patients for hospital admissions: evaluation of a pilot programme for day cases'. *British Medical Journal*, vol 327, pp 1147–52.

Meredith P, Ham C, Kipping R (1999). *Modernising the NHS: Booking patients for hospital care first interim report from the evaluation of the National Booked Admissions Programme*. Birmingham: Health Services Management Centre, University of Birmingham.

Milburn A (2002). *Redefining the National Health Service*. Speech to New Health Network. London: Department of Health.

Murray M (2000). 'Patient care: access'. *British Medical Journal*, vol 320, pp 1994–95.

National Audit Office (2005). *Patient Choice at the Point of Referral*. London: The Stationery Office.

National Audit Office (2004). *Tackling Cancer in England: Saving more lives*. London: The Stationery Office.

National Audit Office (2003). *Hip Replacements: An update*. London: The Stationery Office.

National Audit Office (2001a). *Inpatient and Outpatient Waiting in the NHS*. London: The Stationery Office.

National Audit Office (2001b). *Inappropriate Adjustments to NHS Waiting Lists*. London: The Stationery Office.

National Audit Office (1997). *Cataract Surgery in Scotland*. London: The Stationery Office.

NHS Executive (2000). *A Step-By-Step Guide to Improving Outpatient Services: Variations in NHS outpatient performance*. Leeds: Department of Health.

NHS Executive (1999a). *£20 million boost to reduce waiting lists and waiting times*. Press Release 1999/0097. Leeds: Department of Health.

NHS Executive (1999b). *NHS waiting lists and times performance fund*. Health Service Circular 1999/190. Leeds: Department of Health.

NHS Executive (1998a). *Additional resources in 1998/99 to reduce NHS waiting lists*. Health Service Circular 1998/067. Leeds: Department of Health.

NHS Executive (1998b). *The New NHS: Modern and dependable – a national framework for assessing performance*. Leeds: Department of Health.

NHS Executive (1998c). *Additional money for patient care this winter*. Health Services Circular HSC 1998/209. Leeds: Department of Health.

NHS Executive (1997). *Priorities and Planning Guidance for the NHS 1998/99*. Leeds: Department of Health.

NHS Executive (1996). *Priorities and Planning Guidance for the NHS 1997/98*. Leeds: Department of Health.

NHS Health Operational Intelligence Project (2002). *Information for Action: A good practice guide on anticipatory management in healthcare*. Leeds: Department of Health.

NHS Modernisation Agency (2004a). *10 High Impact Changes for Service Improvement and Delivery*. London: Department of Health.

NHS Modernisation Agency (2004b). *Full Evaluation of the 4th Wave 'Moving to Mainstream'*. London: Department of Health.

NHS Modernisation Agency (2003). *The Little Wizard*. London: Department of Health.

NHS Modernisation Agency (2002a). *Evaluation of 3rd Wave National Booking Programme: Summary report*. London: Department of Health.

NHS Modernisation Agency (2002b). *Improving Orthopaedic Services*. London: Department of Health.

NHS Modernisation Agency (various years). *NHS Beacons Learning Handbook*. London: Department of Health.

NHS Modernisation Agency and NHS Confederation (2004). *Breaking the Rules: Is capacity the problem?* London: NHS Confederation.

National Patients' Access Team (2001a). *Moving to Mainstream: 4th wave National Booked Admissions Programme*. Leicester: Department of Health.

National Patients' Access Team (2001b). *The Cancer Services Collaborative Twelve Months On.* Leicester: Department of Health.

National Patients' Access Team (1999). *Annual Report 1999/2000.* Leicester: National Patients' Access Team.

North Central London Strategic Health Authority (2004). *Royal National Orthopaedic Hospital Waiting List Inquiry Report.* London: North Central London Strategic Health Authority.

Ovretveit J, Bate P, Cleary P, Cretin S, Gustafson D, McInnes K, McLeod H, Molfenter T, Plsek P, Robert G, Shortell S, Wilson T (2002). 'Quality collaboratives: lessons from research'. *Quality and Safety in Health Care*, vol 11, pp 345–51.

Parkin D, Dimakou S, Devlin S, Appleby J (2005). *The Impact of Government Targets on Waiting Times for Elective Surgery: New insights from time-to-event analysis.* Paper presented at International Health Economics Association Conference, Barcelona, 2005.

Plumridge N (2005). 'On suspicious minds'. *Health Service Journal*, 5 May, p 15.

Pope V, Sykes PA (2003). 'The forgotten wait: official waiting times often misleading'. *Clinical Governance: An International Journal*, vol 8, 2, pp 109–11.

Powell E (1976). *A New Look at Medicine and Politics: 1975 and after.* London: Pitman.

Reid J (2003). *Choice Speech to the New Health Network.* London: Department of Health.

Robb PJ (2002). 'Surgeons cannot do it all by themselves: they need other staff and resources too'. *Health Service Journal*, 31 January.

Robert G, McLeod H, Ham C (2003). *Modernising Cancer Services: An evaluation of phase 1 of the Cancer Services Collaborative.* Birmingham: Health Services Management Centre, University of Birmingham.

Robert G, McLeod H, Ham C (undated). *Summary Lessons from Phase 1 of the Cancer Services Collaborative.* Birmingham: Health Services Management Centre, University of Birmingham.

Robinson D, Bell CJM, Moller H, Basnet I (2003). 'Effects of the UK Government's 2-week target on waiting times in women with breast cancer in south-east England'. *British Journal of Cancer*, vol 89, 3, pp 492–96.

Rogers H, Warner J, Steyn R, Silvester K, Pepperman M, Nash R (2002). 'Mathematical models miss the point'. *British Medical Journal*, vol 324, p 1336.

Royal College of Radiologists (2002). *Clinical Radiology: A workforce in crisis.* London: Royal College of Radiologists.

Royal College of Radiologists (1998). *A National Audit of Waiting Times for Radiotherapy.* London: Royal College of Radiologists.

Royal College of Surgeons of England (2005a). *Developing a Modern Surgical Workforce.* London: Royal College of Surgeons of England.

Royal College of Surgeons of England (2005b). *Number of surgeons: a crisis waiting to happen.* Press Notice 2005/0001. London: Royal College of Surgeons of England.

Royal Commission on the NHS (1979). *Final Report.* London: Her Majesty's Stationery Office.

Saleh KJ, Wood KC, Gafni A, Gross AE (1997). 'Immediate surgery versus waiting list policy in revision total hip arthroplasty'. *Journal of Arthroplasty*, vol 12, 1, pp 1–10.

Sanders D, Coulter A, McPherson K (1989). *Variations in Hospital Admission Rates: A review of the literature*. London: King's Fund.

Secretary of State for Health (2004). *Autumn Performance Report 2004*. London: The Stationery Office.

Serco Health (2004). *Review of NHS 'Fee for Service' Pilot Programme*. London: Serco Health.

Siciliani L, Hurst J (2003a). *Tackling Excessive Waiting Times for Elective Surgery: A comparative analysis of policies in 12 OECD countries*. Paris: OECD.

Siciliani L, Hurst J (2003b). *Explaining Waiting Times for Elective Surgery Across OECD Countries*. Paris: OECD.

Smith T (1994). 'Waiting times: monitoring the total post-referral wait'. *British Medical Journal*, vol 309, pp 593–96.

Taylor R, Pringle M, Coupland C (2004). *Implications of Offering Patient Choice for Routine Adult Surgical Referrals*. Nottingham: University of Nottingham.

The Sunday Times (2002). 'Secret NHS Waiting Lists Conceal 250,000 Patients'. *The Sunday Times*, 5 May.

Timmins N (2004a). 'Private patients "likely to return to NHS"'. *Financial Times*, 26 June.

Timmins N (2004b). 'Under the knife: why investment in the NHS means radical surgery for the private healthcare sector'. *Financial Times*, 12 June.

Timmins N (2003a). 'NHS use of independent hospitals has hardly risen'. *Financial Times*, 3 April.

Timmins N (2003b). 'Private hospital group offers to clear NHS waiting lists'. *Financial Times*, 8 October.

Waiting List Action Team (1999). *Getting Patients Treated*. London: Department of Health.

Wanless D (2002). *Securing Our Future Health: Taking a long-term view*. London: HM Treasury.

Yates J (1987). *Why Are We Waiting?* Oxford: Oxford University Press.

### Cutting NHS Waiting Times: Identifying strategies for sustainable reductions
*John Appleby*

Waiting times for NHS treatment are at an all-time low, but some areas have been more successful in meeting the challenging targets than others. This research summary outlines recent King's Fund work on waiting times for the Department of Health. It looks at the work carried out by three groups of hospitals: those that have sustained reductions, those with variable performance, and those with a poor record. Drawing on interviews with clinicians and managers, it identifies factors that separate successful from unsuccessful NHS trusts. Finally, it makes recommendations for ways forward.

February 2005, 8 pages, £3.00
Free download at www.kingsfund.org.uk/publications

### Sustaining Reductions in Waiting Times: Identifying successful strategies
*John Appleby, Seán Boyle, Nancy Devlin, Mike Harley, Anthony Harrison, Louise Locock, Ruth Thorlby*

This working paper brings together the findings and conclusions of recent King's Fund work on waiting times, supported by the Department of Health. The research aimed to isolate factors leading to sustainable reductions in waiting times, quantify the impact of waiting times targets on clinical treatment priorities, and identify key information requirements for hospitals in order to reduce inpatient waiting times.

January 2005, 128 pages, £5.00
Free download at www.kingsfund.org.uk/publications

### Access to Elective Care – What should really be done about waiting lists
*Anthony Harrison and Bill New*

Waiting lists have been a feature of non-urgent or 'elective' care ever since the NHS was founded. Over the years there have been various attempts to reduce them, but the lists have continued to grow. Numbers have been reduced under the current Labour government, but some indications suggest that this may be only a temporary reprieve. This publication argues that it is unrealistic to expect waiting lists to disappear altogether. Instead, it argues, the focus must be on managing them better. It proposes a points system used by hospital specialists in New Zealand to decide who should receive priority treatment, based on the severity of patients' symptoms.

February 2000, ISBN 185717299 X, 140 pages, £12.99